Oncology Pocket Guide to Chemotherapy

Oncology Pocket Guide to Chemotherapy

LORRAINE BALTZER, RN, MSN, OCN
Clinical Research Nurse IV
Department of Clinical Research Nursing
Memorial Sloan-Kettering Cancer Center, New York
As of February 7, 1994
Coordinator of Clinical Research Nurses
Department of Hematology/Oncology
St. Elizabeth's Medical Center of Boston
Brighton, Massachusetts

REGINA BERKERY, RN, MSN, OCN
Clinical Nurse Specialist
Department of Clinical Research Nursing
Memorial Sloan-Kettering Cancer Center
New York, New York

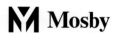 Mosby

St. Louis Baltimore Bogota Boston Buenos Aires Caracas Carlsbad
Chicago London Madrid Mexico City Milan Naples
New York Philadelphia Sydney Tokyo Toronto

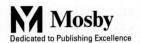
Mosby
Dedicated to Publishing Excellence

Preface

Oncology nurses and physicians play a critical role in the delivery and management of proficient care to cancer patients and their families. Registered nurses are actively involved in the diagnosis, physical and psychologic assessment, treatment, symptom management, and supportive care of patients as they move along the health-illness continuum. Crucial to oncology practice is knowledge of chemotherapeutic agents. Oncology nurses are directly involved in the pharmacologic treatment of cancer and symptom management of side effects and toxicities. This educational pocket guide focuses on the pharmacology, administration, and disposal of specific chemotherapeutic agents. In addition this book highlights the management of chemotherapy-induced side effects.

This *Oncology Pocket Guide to Chemotherapy* is an attempt to condense vital information into a reference book for oncology nurses, physicians, and pharmacists caring for patients receiving chemotherapy. Because of the large number of anticancer agents and space limitations, we have chosen the most widely prescribed conventional agents. We have provided references and bibliographies throughout the book to assist the reader in obtaining further information. It is our hope this book will be helpful to oncology health care professionals in a variety of clinical settings.

Acknowledgements

We wish to thank our loving parents, family, and dedicated colleagues for their support and forbearance during the development of this book. We would like to acknowledge Patricia Bushey for her editorial expertise and Peggy Davis for her assistance in the preparation of portions of this manuscript. We also wish to extend our gratitude to David K. Marshall and Mosby for giving us the opportunity to develop this *Oncology Pocket Guide to Chemotherapy*.

Ms. Baltzer extends a special thanks to Paul D. Cleri for his enduring patience and constant encouragement in the publication of this book. We wish to dedicate this book to our nephews: Maxwell, Christopher, Billy, John, Chris, Matthew, Tommy, Michael, Conor, and Bobbie.

Disclaimer

The drug information presented in this pocket guide was compiled from published reference sources and pharmaceutical package inserts. The authors have made every effort to ensure that information and dosage regimens presented are accurate at the time of publication.

As a result of ongoing research, clinical experience, and changes in government regulations, the authors ask that the reader not use this book as a sole source of chemotherapy drug information; consult primary references, drug information material detailed in package inserts, a pharmacist, and institutional guidelines before administering any agent.

In no case can the authors or the publisher be held responsible for any liability, loss, injury, or damage incurred as a consequence, directly or indirectly, from the use and application of any of the contents of this book. The ultimate responsibility lies with the health care professional on the basis of his or her professional license, experience, and knowledge of the patient to determine the correct dosage and delivery of a drug and the best course of treatment for the patient.

Contents

CHAPTER 3
*Management of
Chemotherapy-Induced Side Effects 151*

*Appendix
Key to FDA Use-In-Pregnancy Ratings 169*

CHAPTER 1

Preparation, Administration, and Disposal of Chemotherapeutic Agents

The preparation, administration, and disposal of chemotherapeutic agents requires a specialized, skilled, and highly knowledgeable professional practice. Registered nurses are routinely responsible for the proper administration of chemotherapeutic agents. It is imperative that the licensed professional administering the chemotherapeutic agent is (1) knowledgeable about the specific agent's mode of administration, mechanism of action, method of metabolism and excretion, indications for usage, and potential adverse effects; (2) has exceptional technical skills in venipuncture and management of venous access devices; and (3) is competent in the safe proper handling and disposal of chemotherapy waste. In addition, any individual administering chemotherapy must be proficient in providing patient and family education.

Prior to the administration of any chemotherapeutic agent, a baseline patient profile, including assessment of the patient's physical, psychological, social, and cognitive status, must be obtained. Following is an outline of prechemotherapy assessment guidelines.*

I. Physical
  A. Past medical history
    1. Cancer diagnosis and history
    2. Previous medical and surgical history
    3. Current medical and surgical problems

    4. Allergies
- B. Laboratory data
  1. Complete blood count including granulocyte/neutrophil count
  2. Platelet count
  3. Other hematopoietic function, if indicated
  4. Liver function
  5. Renal function
- C. System review
  1. Cardiovascular function
  2. Dental and oral cavity status
  3. Dermatologic status
  4. Gastrointestinal function
  5. Neurologic function
  6. Respiratory function
  7. Sexual function
  8. Urologic function
- D. Prior cancer therapy toxicity
  1. Surgery
  2. Chemotherapy
  3. Radiation therapy
  4. Biological therapy

II. Psychologic and social assessment
- A. Life stage development
- B. Previous experience with chemotherapy
- C. Informed consent
- D. Fears
- E. Anxiety
- F. Depression
- G. Intrapersonal resources: coping
- H. Interpersonal resources: social support

III. Educational needs of patient and family
- A. Drug treatment protocol
- B. Potential side effects/adverse reactions
- C. Posttreatment care

---

*Sources: Burke et al., 1991, Holland 1990, Oncology Nursing Society 1988, Rowland 1990. From: Prechemotherapy assessment. In Dorr RT, Von Hoff DD, eds. *Cancer chemotherapy handbook*, 2nd edition. Norwalk, Conn: Appleton & Lange; 1994:58. Reprinted with permission.

Most often chemotherapy dosages are calculated based on the patient's body surface area, expressed in milligrams per square meter, based on the patient's height and weight. Actual heights and weights should be obtained before the administration of every course of chemotherapy. The presence of edema or ascites must be considered so that the dosage will be based on actual weight unaugmented by these conditions. The body surface area is most often calculated by using a nomogram. Figure 1-1 can be used for calculating adult body surface area and Figure 1-2 can be used for calculating a child's body surface area. There is no concrete agreement in the medical community about whether the patient's actual or ideal weight should be used to calculate the proper dosage.

Chemotherapy is administered by systemic or regional modes of delivery. Systemic therapy is aimed at the attainment of a maximal therapeutic cytotoxic effect without extreme toxicity to normal tissues. Systemic chemotherapy is given orally, intravenously, subcutaneously, intramuscularly, or intraosseously. Regional chemotherapy is aimed at delivering chemotherapeutic drugs directly into the blood vessel supplying the tumor or the cavity in which the tumor is located. Intrathecal, intraarterial, and intracavitary routes are used to deliver regional chemotherapy. Regardless of the route of administration, it is imperative that the health care provider delivering chemotherapeutic agents follow specific guidelines for safe handling and disposal of these agents.

The issue of safe handling of hazardous wastes must be addressed in all health care settings. Various organizations have issued guidelines to assist institutions in establishing safe practice policies that utilize optimal protective techniques, thereby limiting exposure to workers. To ensure optimal quality of care and patient safety, specific guidelines have been developed for the safe handling and disposal of antineoplastic agents. These guidelines follow on page 6.

Fig. 1-1 Nomogram for Determining Body Surface of Adults from Height and Weight*

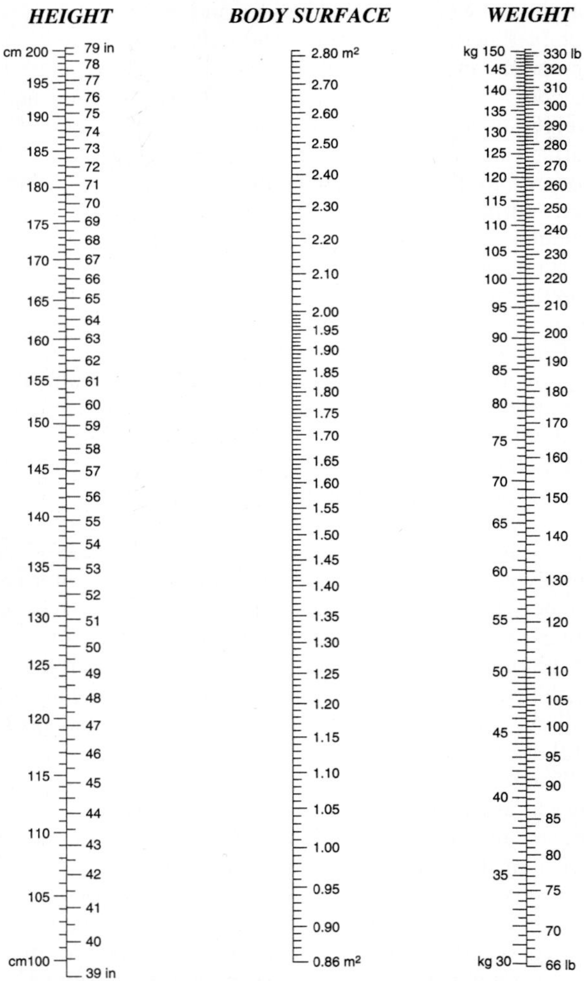

*From the formula of Du Bois and Du Bois, Modified from *Arch. Intern. Med.* 17:863, 1916 ($S = W^{0.425} \times H^{0.725} \times 71.84$, or $\log S = \log W \times 0.425 + \log H \times 0.725 + 1.8564$ [S = body surface in cm^2; W = weight in kg; H = height in cm]).

Fig. 1-2 Nomogram for Determining Body Surface of Children from Height and Weight*

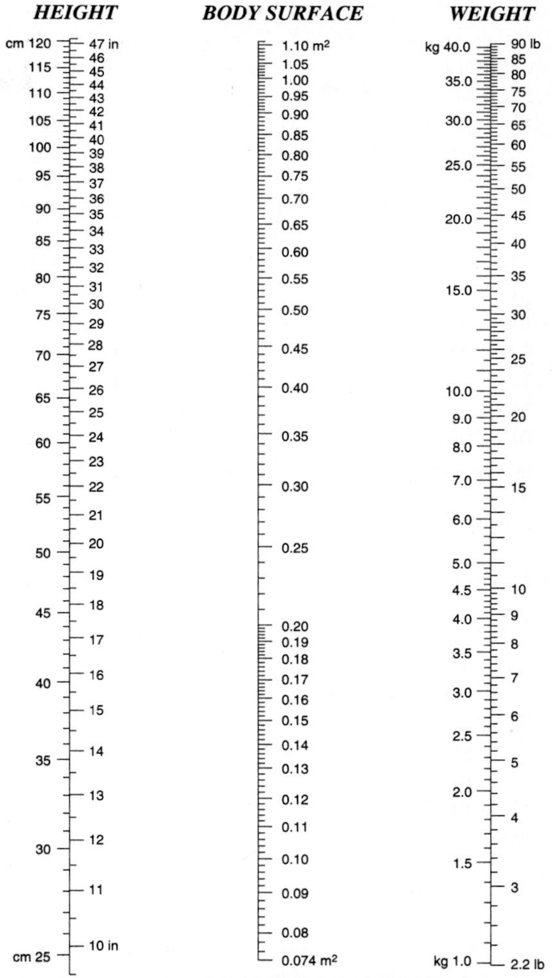

HEIGHT	BODY SURFACE	WEIGHT

*From the formula of Du Bois and Du Bois, Modified from *Arch. Intern. Med.* 17:863, 1916 ($S = W^{0.425} \times H^{0.725} \times 71.84$, or log $S =$ log $W \times 0.425 +$ log $H \times 0.725 + 1.8564$ [$S =$ body surface in cm^2; $W =$ weight in kg; $H =$ height in cm]).

Drug Preparation*

1. All antineoplastic drugs should be prepared by specially trained individuals in a centralized area to minimize interruptions and risk of contamination.

2. Drugs are prepared in a class II biologic safety cabinet (vertical laminar airflow hood) with vents to the outside, if possible. The blower is left on 24 hours a day, 7 days a week. The hood is serviced regularly according to the manufacturer's recommendations.

3. Eating, drinking, smoking, and applying cosmetics in the drug preparation area are prohibited.

4. The work surface is covered with a plastic absorbent pad to minimize contamination. This pad is changed immediately in the event of contamination and at the completion of drug preparation each day or shift.

5. The prescribed drug is prepared using aseptic technique according to the physician's orders, other pharmaceutic resources, or both.

6. Disposable surgical latex unpowdered gloves are used when handling the drugs. Gloves should be changed hourly or immediately if torn or punctured.

7. A disposable long-sleeved gown made of lint-free fabric with knitted cuffs and a closed front is worn during drug preparation.

8. A thermoplastic (Plexiglass®) face shield or goggles and a powered air-purifying respirator should be used if a biologic safety cabinet is not available.

9. Because exposure can result when connecting and disconnecting intravenous (IV) tubing, when injecting the drug into the IV line, when removing air from the syringe or infusion line, and when leakage occurs at the tubing, syringe, or stopcock connection, priming of all IV tubing is carried out under the protection of the hood.

10. Other measures to guard against drug leakage during drug preparation include venting the vial and using large-bore needles, Luer-lock fittings, and sterile gauze or sponge around the neck of the vial during needle withdrawal. Aerosolization may also be minimized by attaching an aerosol protection device

(CytoGuard, Bristol-Myers) to the vial of drug before adding the diluent.

11. Once reconstituted, the drug is labeled according to institutional policies and procedures; the label should include the drug's vesicant properties and antineoplastic drug warning.

12. Antineoplastic drugs are transported in an impervious packing material and are marked with a distinctive warning label.

13. Personnel responsible for drug transport are knowledgeable of procedures to be followed in the event of drug spillage.

Drug Administration*

1. Chemotherapeutic agents are administered by registered professional nurses who have been specially trained and designated as qualified according to specific institutional policies and procedures.

2. Before administering the drugs, the nurse ensures that informed consent has been given and clarifies any misconceptions the patient might have regarding the drugs and their side effects.

3. Appropriate laboratory results are evaluated and found to be within acceptable levels (e.g., complete blood count, renal and liver function).

4. Measures to minimize side effects of the drugs are carried out before drug administration (e.g., hydration, antiemetics and antianxiety agents, and patient comfort).

5. An appropriate route for drug administration is ensured according to the physician's order.

6. Personal protective equipment is worn, including disposable latex surgical gloves and a disposable gown made of a lint-free, low-permeability fabric with a closed front, long sleeves, and elastic or knit closed cuffs (optional).

7. The work surface is protected with a disposable absorbent pad.

8. The drug or drugs are administered according to established institutional policies and procedures.

9. Documentation of drug administration, including

any adverse reaction, is made in the patient's medical record.

10. A mechanism for identification of patients receiving antineoplastic agents is established for the 48-hour period following drug dispensing.

11. Disposable surgical unpowdered latex gloves and a disposable gown are worn when handling body secretions such as blood, vomitus, or excreta from patients who received chemotherapy drugs within the previous 48 hours.

12. In the event of accidental exposure, contaminated gloves and gown should be removed immediately and discarded according to official procedures.

13. Wash the contaminated skin with soap and water.

14. An eye that is accidentally exposed to chemotherapy should be flooded with water or isotonic eyewash for at least 5 minutes.

15. A medical evaluation must be obtained as soon as possible after exposure and the incident documented according to institutional policies and procedures.

Drug Disposal*

1. Regardless of the setting (hospital, ambulatory care, or home), all equipment and unused drugs are treated as hazardous and are disposed of according to the institution's policies and procedures.

2. All contaminated equipment, including needles, are disposed of intact to prevent aerosolization, leaks, and spills.

3. All contaminated materials used in drug preparation are disposed of in a leakproof, punctureproof container with a distinctive warning label and are placed in a sealable 4-mil polyethylene or 2-mil polypropylene bag with appropriate labeling.

4. Linen contaminated with bodily secretions of patients who have received chemotherapy within the previous 48 hours is placed in a specially marked laundry bag, which is then placed in an impervious bag that is marked with a distinctive warning label.

5. In the event of a spill, personnel should don double surgical latex unpowdered gloves; eye protection; and a disposable gown made of a lint-free, low-

permeability fabric with a closed front, long sleeves, and elastic or knit closed cuffs.

6. Small amounts of liquids are cleaned up with gauze pads, whereas larger spills (more than 5 ml) are cleaned up with absorbent pads.

7. Small amounts of solids or spills involving powder are cleaned up with damp cloths or absorbent gauze pads.

8. The spill area is cleaned three times with a detergent followed by clean water.

9. Broken glassware and disposable contaminated materials are placed in a leakproof, punctureproof container and then placed in sealable 4-mil polyethylene or 2-mil polypropylene bag and marked with a distinctive warning label.

10. Contaminated reusable items are washed by specially trained personnel wearing double surgical unpowdered latex gloves.

11. The spill should be documented according to established institutional policies and procedures.

*From: Guidelines for safe handling and disposal of antineoplastic agents. From Goodman M: Delivery of cancer chemotherapy. In Baird SB, McCorkle R, Grant M, eds. *Cancer nursing: a comprehensive textbook.* Philadelphia: WB Saunders; 1991:291-320. Reprinted with permission.

Chemotherapy should be administered only by registered nurses or physicians who are trained in chemotherapy administration. Qualified individuals need to be knowledgeable about the signs and symptoms of extravasation, drugs which have vesicant and irritant properties (Table 1-1), administration techniques of vesicants (Table 1-2), and the recommended extravasation antidotes (Table 1-3). The management of chemotherapy extravasations remains controversial. It is recommended that the reader follow institutional guidelines for the management of specific extravasations.

Table 1-1 Vesicant and Irritant Chemotherapy Agents

VESICANT	*IRRITANT*
Dactinomycin-D	Bleomycin
Daunorubicin HCl	Carboplatin
Doxorubicin HCl	Cisplatin
Idarubicin	Cyclophosphamide
Mechlorethamine HCl	Dacarbazine
Mitomycin-C	Etoposide
Vinblastine	5-Flourouracil
Vincristine	Ifosfamide
	Melphalan
	Mitoxantrone HCl
	Paclitaxel
	Pentostatin
	Streptozocin

Table 1-2 Administration of Vesicant Agents

TWO-SYRINGE TECHNIQUE

1. Select an appropriate vein.
2. Begin a new intravenous line using a scalp vein needle (25- or 23-gauge).
3. Access vein using a single approach.
4. Flush line with 8 to 10 ml of saline. Assess for brisk, full blood return and any evidence of infiltration. Check for swelling, redness, or pain at the site, and lack of blood return.
5. Once access is ensured, switch to syringe of chemotherapy.
6. Dilute drugs according to the package insert.
7. Inject drugs slowly and with minimal resistance.
8. Assess for blood return every 1 to 2 ml of infusion.

SIDEARM TECHNIQUE

1. Ensure proper venous access site. The intravenous fluid should be additive-free.
2. The cannula used to access the vein should be at least a 20-gauge to ensure an adequate blood return and fluid flow.
3. Secure cannula but do not obstruct entrance site.
4. Pinch off tubing and assess for blood return.
5. Test the vein with 50 to 100 ml to ensure an adequate and swift drip of infusion.
6. With intravenous fluid continuing to drip, slowly inject vesicant into intravenous line.
7. Do not allow vesicant to flow backward.
8. Do not pinch off tubing except to assess for blood return.
9. Assess for blood return every 1 or 2 ml of injection.
10. Flush needle with saline at the completion of injection.

From Goodmen M. Delivery of cancer chemotherapy. In: Baird SB, McCorkle R, Grant M, eds. *Cancer nursing: a comprehensive textbook.* Philadelphia: WB Saunders; 1991: 291-320. Reprinted with permission.

Table 1-3 Recommended Extravasation Antidotes

CLASS/SPECIFIC AGENTS	LOCAL ANTIDOTE RECOMMENDED
Alkylating agents Cisplatin[a], Mechlorethamine HCl	1/6 or 1/3 M sodium thiosulfate
Mitomycin-C	Dimethylsulfoxide 50%-99%(w/v) solution
DNA intercalators Doxorubicin HCl Daunorubicin HCl	Cold compresses
Amsacrine[b]	Dimethylsulfoxide 50%-99% (w/v) solution
Vinca alkaloids Vinblastine Vincristine	Warm compresses, Hyaluronidase
Epipodophyllotoxins[a] Etoposide, Teniposide	Warm compresses, Hyaluronidase

[a]Treatment indicated only for large extravasations (e.g., doses one-half or more of the planned total dose for that course of therapy).

[b]Amsacrine is an investigational agent.

From: Recommended extravasation antidotes. In Dorr RT, Von Hoff DD, ed. *Cancer chemotherapy handbook*, 2nd edition. Norwalk, Connecticut: Appleton and Lange; 1994: 115. Reprinted with permission.

SPECIFIC PROCEDURE

Mix 4-8 ml 10% sodium thiosulfate USP with 6 ml of sterile water for injection, USP for a 1/6 or 1/3 M solution. Inject 2 ml into site for each milligram of mechlorethamine or 100 mg of cisplatin extravasated.

Apply 1.5 ml to the site every 6 hours for 14 days. Allow to air-dry; do not cover.

Apply immediately for 30-60 minutes, then alternate off/on every 15 minutes for 1 day.

Apply 1.5 ml to the site every 6 hours for 14 days. Allow solution to air-dry; do not cover.

Apply immediately for 30-60 minutes, then alternate off/on every 15 minutes for 1 day. Inject 150 U hyaluronidase (Wydase, others) into site.

Apply immediately for 30-60 minutes, then alternate off/on every 15 minutes for 1 day. Inject 150 U hyaluronidase (Wydase®, others) into site.

Anaphylactic, allergic, and hypersensitive reactions can result from overstimulation of the immune system during and after the administration of chemotherapy. The following list describes recommended procedures to be taken in the prevention and treatment of hypersensitivity and anaphylactic reactions as outlined by the Oncology Nursing Society:*

1. Review the patient's allergy history and record baseline blood pressure, pulse, and respiration.
2. Consider prophylactic medication with hydrocortisone or an antihistamine in individuals with suspected hypersensitivity potential (this requires a physician's order).
3. Inform the patient of the potential for hypersensitivity reaction and the necessity to report any of the following symptoms immediately:
   a. Urticaria.
   b. Localized/generalized itching.
   c. Shortness of breath with or without wheezing.
   d. Uneasiness or agitation.
   e. Periorbital or facial edema.
   f. Light-headedness/dizziness.
   g. Tightness in the chest.
   h. Abdominal cramping.
   i. Chills.
4. Ensure that emergency equipment (e.g., oxygen, AMBU bag, intubation equipment) is readily available and that there is a patent IV line; check the supply of the following drugs and be familiar with appropriate doses and routes:
   a. Epinephrine.
   b. Diphenhydramine HCl or other antihistamines.
   c. Hydrocortisone sodium succinate.
   d. Aminophylline.
   e. Dopamine HCl.
   f. Dexamethasone.
5. Before administering the initial dose of a drug with reports of increased incidence of hypersensitivity, a scratch test, intradermal skin test, or test dose may be performed first (all of these procedures require a physician's order):

    a. Observe the patient for at least 15 minutes after the test dose for a local positive reaction and/or a systemic reaction; if positive, notify the physician. A systemic reaction can occur up to an hour after the test dose.

    b. If no signs of hypersensitivity response occur, precede with initial dosing.

    c. If administering drug by intravenous infusion, give slowly and observe patient closely for additional 25 minutes.

    d. If a hypersensitivity response is suspected, discontinue infusion of drug, maintain the intravenous line, administer emergency drugs if preordered, and notify the physician.

6. For a localized hypersensitivity response:

    a. Observe and evaluate symptoms: urticaria, wheals, localized erythema.

    b. Administer diphenhydramine and/or hydrocortisone according to the physician's order.

    c. Monitor vital signs every 15 minutes for 1 hour.

    d. If patient is considered sensitized, avoid subsequent dosing. However, if drug is critical in treatment plan, premedication with antihistamines and corticosteroids may prevent a hypersensitivity response; a desensitization program may be indicated.

    e. If a flare reaction appears along the vein with doxorubicin or daunorubicin, stop the drug and flush the vein with saline.

        i. Assess for immediate manifestation of extravasation to determine if this is a flare reaction or extravasation.

        ii. If extravasation is not suspected, continue with saline flush and observe for resolution of flare reaction.

        iii. If resolution does not occur, administer hydrocortisone, 25-50 mg, and/or diphenhydramine, 25-50 mg, intravenously with a physician's order, followed by saline flush.

        iv. Once the flare reaction has resolved,

resume infusion of the drug at a much slower rate.

v. Monitor for repeated flare episodes; it may be preferable to change the intravenous site.

vi. If the drug is to be readministered at a later date, consider premedication with antihistamines and glucocorticoids; slower infusion rates and/or greater fluid volumes also may be helpful.

7. For a generalized hypersensitivity/anaphylactic response, suspect, if any or all of the following signs/symptoms occur (usually within the first 15 minutes from start of infusion/injection):

a. Subjective signs/symptoms:
   i. Generalized itching.
   ii. Chest tightness.
   iii. Agitation.
   iv. Dizziness.
   v. Nausea.
   vi. Cramps/abdominal pain.
   vii. Anxiety.
   viii. Chills.
   ix. Burning/tingling sensations.

b. Objective signs/symptoms:
   i. Localized or generalized urticaria.
   ii. Flushed appearance (angioedema of face, neck, eyelids, hands, and feet).
   iii. Respiratory distress with or without wheezing.
   iv. Hypotension.
   v. Cyanosis.

c. Management:
   i. Immediate action is imperative; many actions may need to be performed simultaneously.
   ii. Stop chemotherapy injection/infusion immediately.
   iii. Stay with patient; another staff member should notify physician.
   iv. Maintain intravenous line with normal saline or another appropriate solution to

expand vascular space.
v. Administer emergency drugs according to standing orders or physician's order: epinephrine, 0.1-0.5 mg (1:10,000 solution) intravenous push, repeat every 10 minutes as needed; pediatric dose is 0.01 mg/kg; adult subcutaneous epinephrine (1:1000 solution) doses are 0.2-0.5 mg; pediatric patients can receive 0.01 mg/kg; subcutaneous doses may be repeated every 10-15 minutes if needed.
vi. Place patient in supine position.
vii. Monitor vital signs every 2 minutes until stable, every 5 minutes for 30 minutes, then every 15 minutes until stable.
viii. Maintain patient's airway, assessing for increasing edema of the respiratory passageway. Administer oxygen if needed. Anticipate the need for cardiopulmonary resuscitation.
ix. Reassure patient and family.
x. Administer other emergency drugs as needed:
    (1) Antihistamines such as diphenhydramine HCl (Benadryl®) 25-50 mg intravenously to block further antigen-antibody reaction.
    (2) Adrenal steroids such as Solu-Medrol® 30-60 mg IV or Solu Cortef® 100-500 mg IV or dexamethasone 10-20 mg intravenously, to ease bronchoconstriction and cardiac dysfunction.
    (3) Aminophylline 5 mg/kg over 30 minutes intravenously to produce bronchodilation.
    (4) Vasopressors such as dopamine 2-20 μm/kg/min to counter hypotension.
8. Document all treatment in patient's medical record.
9. Avoid using chemotherapy agents causing anaphylaxis/hypersensitivity in the future. If drug is

necessary in treatment plan; however, health care team should consider and discuss the following options:

a. Physician-guided desensitization.
b. Premedication with antihistamines and/or corticosteroids.
c. Additional fluid for drug dilution.
d. Increased infusion time.
e. Substitution of a similar drug (e.g., using *Erwinia* L-asparaginase instead of *E. coli*).

*From Oncology Nursing Society. *Cancer Chemotherapy Guidelines: Recommendations for the management of vesicant extravastion, hypersensitivity and anaphylaxis.* Pittsburgh, PA: Oncology Nursing Society; 1992. Reprinted with permission.

BIBLIOGRAPHY

Baird SB, McCorkle R, Grant M, eds. *Cancer nursing: a comprehensive textbook.* Philadelphia: WB Saunders; 1991.

Burke MB, Wilkes GM, Berg D, Bean CK, Ingwersen K. Principles of chemotherapy administration and drug delivery systems. In: *Cancer chemotherapy: a nursing process approach.* Boston: Jones & Bartlett; 1991: 375-423.

DeVita VT, Hellman S, Rosenberg SA. *Cancer principles and practice of oncology,* 4th edition. Philadelphia: JB Lippincott; 1993.

Dorr RT, Von Hoff DD, eds. *Cancer chemotherapy handbook,* 2nd edition. Norwalk, Conn: Appleton & Lange; 1994.

Groenwald SL, Frogge MF, Goodman M, Yarbro CH. *Cancer nursing principles in practice,* 2nd edition. Boston: Jones & Bartlett; 1992.

Holland JC. Fears and abnormal reactions to cancer in physically healthy individuals. In: Holland JC, Rowland JH, eds. *Handbook of psychooncology: psychological care of the patient with cancer.* New York: Oxford University Press; 1990: 13-21.

Occupational Safety and Health Administration. Work practice guidelines for personnel dealing with cytotoxic (antineoplastic) drugs. *OSHA Instructional Publication 8-1.1* Washington, DC: Office of Occupational Medicine; 1986.

Oncology Nursing Society. *Cancer chemotherapy guidelines: Module I-IV.* Pittsburgh: Oncology Nursing Society; 1992.

Oncology Nursing Society. *Cancer chemotherapy guidelines: recommendations for the management of vesicant extravasation, hypersensitivity and anaphylaxis.* Pittsburgh: Oncology Nursing Society; 1992.

Otto SE. *Oncology nursing.* St. Louis: Mosby; 1991.

Rowland JH. Interpersonal resources: social support and coping. In: Holland JC, Rowland JH, eds. *Handbook of psychooncology: psychological care of the patient with cancer.* New York: Oxford University Press; 1990: 44-71.

CHAPTER 2

Chemotherapeutic Agents

This chapter is designed to give the health care professional brief monographs of common conventional chemotherapeutic agents. Details regarding each agent's synonyms, mechanism of action, metabolism and excretion, FDA-approved and investigational indications, FDA-approved dosing schedules, administration, stability, drug interactions, side effects and toxicities, warnings, precautions, and special considerations are provided. Appendix 1 is a key to "FDA use in pregnancy ratings," which are listed in the drug monographs.

The FDA-approved indications at the time of this publication are highlighted with an asterisk (*). The dosage and schedule of each agent are exactly as prescribed in the manufacture package inserts, which are the FDA-approved recommendations. The Food Drug and Cosmetic Act "does not, however, limit the manner in which a physician may use an approved drug. Once a product has been approved for marketing, a physician may prescribe it for uses or in treatment regimens or patient populations that are not included in the approved labeling." There are a variety of therapeutic dosages and schedules for the chemotherapy agents listed that are not included in the pocket guide related to the lack of current FDA recognition. It is for these reasons we strongly urge the reader to review original published sources for variations in the use, dose, and schedule of all agents.

Selected references for each drug are listed at the end of each monograph. Additionally, a bibliography of the comprehensive chemotherapy references used as data sources is found at the end of the chapter. We ask that the reader NOT use this chapter as the sole source of chemotherapy information; refer to primary literature sources and manufacturer package inserts for current dosing schedules and side effect profiles.

This chapter is offered as a brief reference guide to specific chemotherapeutic agents. Since all drugs used in cancer chemotherapy are potentially hazardous, it is recommended that only those physicians experienced with the risks of the drug, who are fully knowledgeable in the natural history of the malignant disease being treated and the assessment of response to chemotherapy, prescribe any of the drugs found in this pocket guide.

Asparaginase

Elspar®, L-ASP, L-asparaginase

MECHANISM OF ACTION
Asparaginase is an enzyme that inhibits the protein synthesis dependent on asparagine. Asparaginase hydrolyzes asparagine to aspartic acid and ammonia, thereby depleting tumor cells of asparagine.

METABOLISM/EXCRETION
Mild urinary and biliary excretion occurs. Plasma half-life varies from 8-30 hours.

INDICATIONS
1. Acute lymphocytic leukemia* (in combination with other agents in the induction of remissions in children)
2. Chronic myelocytic leukemia
3. Acute myelocytic leukemia

DOSAGE AND SCHEDULE
Adult and Pediatric
Induction regimens: When using chemotherapeutic agents in combination for the induction of remissions in patients with acute lymphocytic leukemia, regimens are sought that provide maximum chance of success while avoiding excessive cumulative toxicity or negative drug interactions. One of the following combination regimens incorporating Elspar is recommended for acute lymphocytic leukemia in children. In the regimens below, day 1 is considered to be the first day of therapy.

Regimen 1:

Prednisone 40 mg/m^2/day PO in 3 divided doses for 15 days, followed by tapering of the dosage as follows: 20 mg/m^2 for 2 days, 10 mg/m^2 for 2 days, 5 mg/m^2 for 2 days, 2.5 mg/m^2 for 2 days, and then discontinue.

Vincristine sulfate 2 mg/m^2 IV once weekly on days 1,8, and 15 of the treatment period. The maximum single dose should not exceed 2 mg.

Asparaginase 1,000 IU/kg/day IV for 10 successive days beginning on day 22 of the treatment period.

Regimen 2:

Prednisone 40 mg/m^2/day PO in 3 divided doses for 28 days (the total daily dose should be to the nearest 2.5 mg), following which the dosage of prednisone should be discontinued gradually over a 14-day period.

Vincristine sulfate 1.5 mg/m^2 IV weekly for 4 doses, on days 1,8,15, and 22 of the treatment period. The maximum single dose should not exceed 2 mg.

Asparaginase 6,000 IU/m^2 IM on days 4,7,10,13,16,19,22,25, and 28 of the treatment period.

When a remission is obtained with either of the above regimens, appropriate maintenance therapy must be instituted. Elspar should not be used as part of a maintenance regimen. The above regimens do not preclude a need for special therapy directed toward the prevention of central nervous system leukemia.

It should be noted that Elspar has been used in combination regimens other than those recommended above. It is important to keep in mind that Elspar administered IV concurrently with or immediately before a course of vincristine and prednisone may be associated with increased toxicity. Physicians using a given regimen should be thoroughly familiar with its benefits and risks. Clinical data are insufficient for a recommendation concerning the use of combination regimens in adults. Asparaginase toxicity is reported to be greater in adults than in children.

Use of Elspar as the sole induction agent should be undertaken only in an unusual situation when a combined regimen is inappropriate because of toxicity or other specific patient-related factors, or in cases refractory to other therapy. When Elspar is to be used as the sole induction agent for children or adults, the recommended dosage regimen is 200 IU/kg/day IV for 28 days. When complete remissions were obtained with this regimen, they were of short duration (1-3 months). Elspar has been used as the sole induction agent in other regimens.

Patients who have received a course of Elspar, if retreated, have an increased risk of hypersensitive reactions. Retreatment should be undertaken only when the benefit of such therapy is weighed against the increased risk.

Intradermal skin test:

Because of the occurrence of allergic reactions, an intradermal skin test should be performed before the initial administration of Elspar and when Elspar is given after an interval of a week or more between doses. The skin test solution may be prepared as follows: Reconstitute the contents of a 10,000 IU vial with 5 ml of diluent. From this solution (2,000 IU/ml) withdraw 0.1 ml and inject it into another vial containing 9.9 ml of diluent, yielding a skin test solution of approximately 20 IU/ml. Use 0.1 ml of this solution (2 IU) for the intradermal skin test. The skin test should be observed for at least 1 hour for the appearance of a wheal or erythema, either of which indicates a positive reaction. An allergic reaction even to the skin test dose in certain sensitized individuals may rarely occur. A negative skin test reaction does not preclude the possibility of the development of an allergic reaction.

ADMINISTRATION

Intravenous over 30 minutes through the side arm of an already running infusion of normal saline or D_5W. *Intramuscular* in a volume not greater than 2 ml for each injection site. *Intradermal skin testing* is recommended before the first dose of asparaginase and repeated if the interval between doses is 7 or more days.

STABILITY

Once reconstituted, asparaginase should be used within 8 hours or it must be discarded.

DRUG INTERACTIONS

- The use of asparaginase concurrently or before a course of prednisone and vincristine may be associated with increased toxicity.
- Asparaginase in combination with prednisone may cause an increase in hyperglycemia.
- Asparaginase administered before vincristine may increase the neurotoxic effects of vincristine.
- Asparaginase may interfere with the cellular uptake of methotrexate.
- Asparaginase may cause an increase in toxicity to other medications because of the adverse effect of asparaginase on liver function.

SIDE EFFECTS AND TOXICITIES

Hematologic

Mild bone marrow suppression (anemia and leukopenia); prolongation of clotting factors (Factors V, VII, VIII, IX, prothrombin, and fibrinogen), fatal bleeding, disseminated intravascular coagulation.

Gastrointestinal

Mild nausea, vomiting, anorexia, abdominal cramps, weight loss, increase in SGOT, SGPT, alkaline phosphatase, and bilirubin, as well as a decrease in serum albumin, cholesterol (total and ester), and plasma fibrinogen; hypoalbuminemia with associated peripheral edema, malabsorption syndrome, pancreatitis (can be fatal), hyperglycemia with glucosuria and polyuria (may respond to insulin and discontinuation of the drug), diabetic ketoacidosis.

Renal

Azotemia, acute renal failure, fatal renal insufficiency, proteinuria, increased serum uric acid levels.

Cardiac

Hypotension.

Neurologic

Depression, fatigue, coma, confusion, agitation, hallucinations, Parkinson-like syndrome with tremors and a progressive increase in muscle tone, increase in blood ammonia levels.

Hypersensitivities

Allergic/anaphylactic reactions: skin rashes, urticaria,

arthralgia, respiratory distress, laryngeal constriction, hypotension, diaphoresis, edema, bronchospasm, loss of consciousness.

Reproductive

There are no adequate studies on the effects of asparaginase on fertility.

Secondary Neoplasias

The drug has possible mutagenic and carcinogenic properties.

Miscellaneous

Fever and chills.

WARNINGS/PRECAUTIONS

- Allergic/anaphylactic reactions may be fatal and can occur with any dose in the presence of a negative skin test. It is recommended that asparaginase be administered only in a hospital setting with treatment readily available in case of allergic/hypersensitive reactions.
- Asparaginase is contraindicated in patients who have had a previous anaphylactic reaction. The investigational form of asparaginase (Erwinia) has been used in patients with allergic reactions to *E. Coli* asparaginase (Elspar). Allergic/anaphylactic reactions may still occur.
- Asparaginase toxicity may be greater in adults than in children.
- Monitor serum amylase to detect early pancreatitis. Asparaginase is contraindicated in patients with pancreatitis or a history of pancreatitis. If pancreatitis develops, discontinue use of asparaginase. Acute hemorrhagic pancreatitis has occurred.
- Monitor liver function tests. Asparaginase has an adverse effect on liver function.
- Asparaginase may interfere with interpretation of thyroid function tests.
- Pregnancy category C. Nursing infants may experience serious adverse reactions from asparaginase.

SPECIAL CONSIDERATIONS

- Monitor the patient during the administration of asparaginase for anaphylaxis.
- Allergic/anaphylactic reactions can occur with either

the IV, IM, or the skin test route and usually respond to the use of epinephrine, oxygen, and steroids.

- An increase in serum uric acid levels may occur when therapy is initiated causing the development of uric acid nephropathy. Preventive measures should be instituted (e.g., allopurinol, urine alkalinization, increased fluid intake).

Selected Readings

Killander D, Dohlwitz A, Engstedt L, et al. Hypersensitivity reactions and antibody formation during L-asparaginase treatment of children and adults with acute leukemia. *Cancer.* 1972;**37**:220-228.

Land VJ, Sutow WW, Fernbach DJ, et al. Toxicity of L-asparaginase in children with advanced leukemia. *Cancer.* 1972;**30**:339-347.

Oettgen HF, Stephenson PA, Schwartz MK, et al. Toxicity of *E. coli* L-asparaginase in man. *Cancer.* 1970;**25**:253-278.

Ramsay NKC, Coccia PF, Krivit W, et al. The effect of L-asparaginase on plasma coagulation factors in acute lymphoblastic leukemia. *Cancer.* 1977;**40**:1398-1401.

Zubrod CG. The clinical toxicities of L-asparaginase in treatment of leukemia and lymphoma. *Pediatrics.* 1970;**45**:555-559.

Bleomycin Sulfate

Blenoxane®, Bleo

MECHANISM OF ACTION
An antitumor antibiotic, bleomycin sulfate inhibits DNA synthesis and may inhibit RNA and protein synthesis. Cell cycle specific.

METABOLISM/EXCRETION
Bleomycin sulfate is rapidly inactivated by the liver and kidneys and excreted primarily by the kidneys. Approximately 50% of the dose is found in the urine.

INDICATIONS
1. Testicular carcinoma: embryonal cell, choriocarcinoma, teratocarcinoma*
2. Lymphomas: Hodgkin's, reticulum cell sarcoma, and lymphosarcoma
3. Squamous cell carcinoma of the head and neck*
4. Squamous cell carcinoma of the skin, cervix, vulva, and penis*

DOSAGE AND SCHEDULE

Because of the possibility of an anaphylactoid reaction, lymphoma patients should be treated with 2 units or less for the first 2 doses. If no acute reaction occurs, then the regular dosage schedule may be followed.

Adult

Squamous cell carcinoma, lymphosarcoma, reticulum cell sarcoma, testicular carcinoma: 0.25-0.50 units/kg (10-20 units/m^2) given IV, IM, or SQ weekly or twice weekly.

Hodgkin's disease: Dosing as above and after a 50% response, a maintenance dose of 1 unit daily or 5 units weekly IV, or IM should be given.

Pulmonary toxicity of Blenoxane appears to be dose-related with a striking incidence when the total dose is over 400 units. Total doses over 400 units should be given with great caution.

Note: When Blenoxane is used in combination with other antineoplastic agents, pulmonary toxicities may occur at lower doses.

ADMINISTRATION

Intravenous slowly over 10 minutes or longer.
Subcutaneous. Intramuscular.

STABILITY

Stable for 24 hours at room temperature in sodium chloride or D$_5$W.

DRUG INTERACTIONS

- The elimination of bleomycin sulfate may be altered and an increase in toxicity may occur when given with other nephrotoxic agents.
- Raynaud's syndrome may occur when bleomycin sulfate is combined with vinblastine.
- Radiation therapy can increase the pulmonary toxic effects of bleomycin.

SIDE EFFECTS AND TOXICITIES

Hematologic

Mild myelosuppression.

Gastrointestinal

Mild nausea, vomiting, and anorexia; decrease in liver function.

Renal
Decrease in renal function; thrombotic microangiopathy.
Pulmonary
Pulmonary toxicity (dose limiting toxicity); signs and symptoms of dyspnea and rales are early indications of bleomycin-induced pulmonary toxicity. The toxicity presents as pneumonitis and progresses to pulmonary fibrosis, which may be fatal. Pulmonary function tests showing a decrease in vital capacity and total lung volume may be indications of pulmonary toxicity.
Cardiac
Chest pain; myocardial infarction reported in patients receiving bleomycin with other chemotherapeutic agents.
Neurologic
Cerebrovascular accidents reported with bleomycin in combination with other drugs; headache and lethargy.
Dermatologic
Hyperpigmentation of skin, erythema, pruritus, stomatitis, alopecia (thinning), increased sensitivity to sunlight, and thickening of the nail beds; dose-related skin toxicity occurring after 150-200 units.
Hypersensitivities
Anaphylaxis; idiosyncratic reactions: hypotension, wheezing, fever, chills, and confusion (delayed onset).
Reproductive
There are no adequate studies on the effects of bleomycin on fertility.
Secondary Neoplasias
The drug may have carcinogenic, teratogenic, and mutagenic properties.
Miscellaneous
Fever and chills.
WARNINGS/PRECAUTIONS
- Contraindicated in patients who have had a hypersensitive or idiosyncratic reaction to bleomycin. Careful monitoring for anaphylaxis is important since it can occur after any dose. Treatment of anaphylactic reactions may include volume expansion, pressor agents, antihistamines, and corticosteroids.
- People who have received bleomycin in their lifetime

must inform their anesthesiologists. The pulmonary toxicity from bleomycin may be enhanced by the high intraoperative FIO_2.

- Higher incidence of pulmonary toxicity occurs in patients > 70 years of age and in patients who have received > 400 units total cumulative dose, although this toxicity has been seen in younger patients and at lower doses.
- Use cautiously in patients with impaired pulmonary function, patients > 70 years old, and patients with impaired renal function. Dose reductions are recommended for impaired renal function.
- Pregnancy category C. It is not known if the drug is excreted in human milk.

SPECIAL CONSIDERATIONS

- Chest x-rays and pulmonary function tests should be done at baseline and throughout treatment to assess for pulmonary toxicity. If the diffusion capacity for carbon monoxide (DL_{co}) decreases by 30% of baseline, bleomycin should be discontinued.

Selected Readings

Blum RH, Carter SK, Agre K. A clinical review of bleomycin—a new, antineoplastic agent. *Cancer.* 1973;**31:**903-914.

Cohen IS, Mosher MB, O'Keefe EJ, et al. Cutaneous toxicity of bleomycin therapy. *Arch Dermatol.* 1973;**107:**553-555.

Crooke ST, Bradner WT. Bleomycin: A review. *J Med.* 1976;**7:**333-428.

Rudders RA, Hensley GT. Bleomycin pulmonary toxicity. *Chest.* 1973;**63:**626-628.

Samuels ML, Holoye PY, Johnson DE. Bleomycin combination chemotherapy in the management of testicular neoplasia. *Cancer.* 1975;**36:**318-326.

Van Barneveld PWC, Sleijfer DT, Van Der Mark TW, et al. Natural course of bleomycin-induced pneumonitis. *Am Rev Respir Dis.* 1987;**135:**48-51.

Yagoda A, Mukherji B, Young C, et al. Bleomycin, an anti-tumor antibiotic. Clinical experience in 274 patients. *Ann Intern Med.* 1972;77:861-870.

Busulfan

Myleran®, BSF, busulphan
MECHANISM OF ACTION
Methanesulfonate-type alkylating agent. Appears to interact with cellular thiol groups and nucleic acids. Cell cycle nonspecific. Busulfan interferes with the biological function of DNA by crosslinking DNA-DNA and DNA-protein.
METABOLISM/EXCRETION
Well absorbed orally. Metabolized by the liver. Metabolites are excreted in the urine, with 10%-50% excreted within 48 hours. Half-life is unknown. The drug crosses the placental barrier.
INDICATIONS
1. Chronic myelogenous (myeloid, granulocytic, myelocytic) leukemia*
2. Bone marrow transplantation for refractory leukemia, lymphomas, and advanced pediatric solid tumors, in high doses with cyclophosphamide
DOSAGE AND SCHEDULE
Adult
Busulfan is administered orally. The usual adult dose range for remission induction is 4-8 mg/day. Dosing on a weight basis is the same for adult and pediatric patients, approximately 6 µg/kg of body weight, or 1.8 mg/m^2 of body surface, daily. Since the rate of fall of the leukocyte count is dose related, daily doses exceeding 4 mg/day should be reserved for patients with the most compelling symptoms; the greater the total daily dose, the greater is the possibility of inducing bone marrow aplasia.

A decrease in the leukocyte count is not usually seen during the first 10-15 days of treatment; the leukocyte count may actually increase during this period and it should not be interpreted as resistance to the drug, nor should the dose be increased. Since the leukocyte count may continue to fall for more than 1 month after discontinuing the drug, it is important that busulfan be discontinued before the total leukocyte count falling into the normal range. When the total leukocyte count has declined to approximately 15,000/mm^3 the drug should be withheld.

With a constant dose of busulfan, the total leukocyte count declines exponentially; a weekly plot of the leukocyte count aids in predicting the time when therapy should be discontinued. With the recommended dose of busulfan, a normal leukocyte count is usually achieved in 12-20 weeks.

During remission, the patient is examined at monthly intervals and treatment resumed with the induction dosage when the total leukocyte count reaches approximately 50,000/mm^3. When remission is shorter than 3 months, maintenance therapy of 1-3 mg/day may be advisable to keep the hematologic status under control and prevent rapid relapse.

Pediatric
The safety and effectiveness in children have not been well established.

ADMINISTRATION
Oral 2 mg scored tablets.

STABILITY
Stable at room temperature (15°-25°C or 59°-77°F).

DRUG INTERACTIONS
- Concomitant use with thioguanine may cause hepatic dysfunction and/or esophageal varices.
- Probenecid and sulfinpyrazone may increase blood and urine uric acid levels.

SIDE EFFECTS AND TOXICITIES
Hematologic
Severe bone marrow depression; thrombocytopenia, leukopenia, pancytopenia, with a nadir in 11-30 days, recovery in 24-54 days. Delayed and refractory pancytopenia may occur and can be lethal. Rare agranulocytosis.

Gastrointestinal
Nausea and vomiting increases with high-dose therapy; diarrhea, cholestatic jaundice, weight loss.

Renal
Hyperuricemia, adrenal insufficiency-like syndrome, flank pain, renal calculi, uric acid nephropathy, acute renal failure.

Pulmonary
Rare bronchopulmonary dysplasia progressing to

irreversible pulmonary fibrosis ("busulfan lung") and pneumonitis may begin 1 to 10 years following therapy (average onset 4 years); corticosteriods may be helpful, but the condition is usually fatal within 6 months of onset, related to rapid, diffuse fibrosis

Cardiac

Endocardial fibrosis

Neurologic

Dizziness

Dermatologic

Alopecia, dermatitis, hyperpigmentation of skin creases from increased melanin production.

Secondary Neoplasias

Mutagenic, teratogenic, and carcinogenic properties

Hypersensitivities

As with all drugs, hypersensitivity, allergic reactions, and anaphylaxis may occur

Reproductive

Impotence, male sterility, amenorrhea (potentially irreversible), gynecomastia, testicular atrophy, azoospermia, ovarian suppression, menopausal symptoms

WARNINGS/PRECAUTIONS

- Contraindicated in men and women of childbearing potential, patients receiving concurrent radiation or chemotherapy, lactating or pregnant women, patients with leukopenia, thrombocytopenia, or anemia, and patients with hepatotoxicity and/or renal toxicity.
- Do not give to patients with known hypersensitivity or in blastic phase chronic myelocytic leukemia.
- Pregnancy category D. It is not known whether the drug is excreted in human milk.

SPECIAL CONSIDERATIONS

- Patients are at risk for hyperuricemia if the WBC is too high; allopurinol and hydration may be necessary.
- Take medication at the same time each day.
- Taking busulfan on an empty stomach may decrease the degree of nausea and vomiting.

Selected Readings

Burns WA, McFarland W, Matthews MJ. Busulphan-induced

pulmonary disease: Report of a case and review of the literature. *Am Rev Respir Dis.* 1970;**101:**408-413.

Diamond I, Anderson MM, McCreadie SR. Transplacental transmission of busulfan (myleran) in a mother with leukemia. Production of fetal malformation and cytomegaly. *Pediatrics.* 1960;**25:**85-90.

Heard BE, Cooke RA. Busulfan lung. *Thorax.* 1968;**23:**187-193

Marcus RE, Goldman M. Convulsions due to high-dose busulphan. *Lancet.* 1984;**2:**1463.

Carboplatin

Paraplatin®, CBDCA

MECHANISM OF ACTION

Cell cycle nonspecific alkylating-like agent. Although the exact mechanism of action is unknown, it is postulated that action is via covalent binding to DNA, intrastrand and interstrand DNA cross-links, and DNA-protein cross-links.

METABOLISM/EXCRETION

There is little if any true metabolism of the drug. Within 24 hours, 70% of the drug is excreted by the kidneys in the urine. Half-life: initial 1-2 hours, postdistribution $2^1/_2$ - 6 hours.

INDICATIONS

1. Ovarian cancer(advanced)*
2. Endometrial carcinoma
3. Non-small cell lung cancer
4. Head and neck cancer
5. Metastatic seminoma
6. Recurrent brain tumors in children
7. Relapsed and refractory acute leukemia

DOSAGE AND SCHEDULE

Aluminum reacts with carboplatin causing precipitate formation and loss of potency; therefore, needles of intravenous sets containing aluminum parts that may come in contact with the drug must not be used for the preparation or administration of Paraplatin.

Adult

Single agent therapy:

Paraplatin as a single agent has been shown to be effective in patients with recurrent ovarian carcinoma at a dosage of 360 mg/m^2 IV on day 1 repeated every 4 weeks. In general, however, single intermittent courses of Paraplatin should not be repeated until the neutrophil count is at least 2,000/mm^3 and the platelet count is at least 100,000/mm^3.

Combination therapy with cyclophosphamide: In the chemotherapy of advanced ovarian cancer, an effective combination for previously untreated patients consists of: Paraplatin—300 mg/m^2 IV on day 1, every 4 weeks for 6 cycles; cyclophosphamide—600 mg/m^2 IV on day 1, every 4 weeks for 6 cycles. Intermittent courses of Paraplatin in combination with cyclophosphamide should not be repeated until the neutrophil count is at least 2,000/mm^3 and the platelet count is at least 100,000/mm^3.

Refer to specific guidelines for dose adjustments for single and combination therapy, modified on the basis of myelosuppression from prior therapy, and for patients with impaired renal function.

Pediatric
Safety and effectiveness have not been established in children.

ADMINISTRATION
Brief *intravenous* infusion over 15-30 minutes or longer with 500 ml of D$_5$W or normal saline. Carboplatin has also been infused intravenously over 1 hour, continuously for 24, 96, and 120 hours, and continuously for 21 days.

STABILITY
Supplied in glass vials containing 50, 150, and 450 mg of drug powder and an equivalent amount of mannitol. Protect from light and store at room temperature (15°-30°C or 59°-86°F). When reconstituted the 10 mg/ml solution is stable for 24 hours. However, discard solution after 8 hours because of lack of bacteriostatic preservative.

DRUG INTERACTIONS
• Increase in ototoxicity and nephrotoxicity when given with aminoglycosides.

SIDE EFFECTS AND TOXICITIES
Hematologic
Myelosuppression is dose-limiting, with a platelet nadir in 14-21 days and recovery by day 28. Leukocyte nadir

occurs 1 week after platelets and recovers in 5-6 weeks. Thrombocytopenia may be severe. Anemia may also prolong therapy.

Gastrointestinal
Nausea and vomiting can be moderate to severe, beginning 6+ hours after initiation and lasting 24 hours. Mild anorexia, diarrhea, constipation, mucositis, alteration in taste perception, weight loss; hepatic dysfunction manifested by changes in alkaline phosphatase, SGOT/SGPT, and bilirubin; hemorrhagic colitis with high-dose therapy.

Renal
Less toxic than cisplatin; hematuria, renal dysfunction, hypermagnesemia, hypocalcemia, hypokalemia, hyponatremia, hyperuremia.

Pulmonary
Interstitial pneumonitis with high-dose therapy.

Cardiotoxic
Cardiac failure, embolism, and cerebrovascular accidents.

Neurologic
Central neurologic toxicities (mild parasthesias), in patients over 65 years of age; patients previously treated with cisplatin, or on prolonged therapy with carboplatin; convulsions, peripheral neuropathies.

Dermatologic
Alopecia, skin rash, skin irritation.

Secondary Neoplasias
The drug is mutagenic and possibly teratogenic.

Hypersensitivities
Hypersensitivity; anaphylactic-like and allergic reactions can occur within minutes of starting the infusion; manifestations include rash, urticaria, erythema, pruritus, rare bronchospasm, and anaphylaxis; flulike syndrome.

Reproductive
Impotence, sterility, amenorrhea, gynecomastia.

Miscellaneous
Ototoxicity: clinical hearing deficits, tinnitus, and decreased audio acuity; optic neuritis with high-dose therapy.

WARNINGS/PRECAUTIONS

- Contraindicated in patients with a history of severe allergic reactions to cisplatin or other platinum-containing compounds, known hypersensitivity, significant bleeding, and bone marrow depression.
- Concomitant use with other drugs that precipitate nephrotoxicity (e.g., aminoglycoside antibiotics) should be given with caution.
- Pregnancy category D. It is not known whether the drug is excreted in human milk.

SPECIAL CONSIDERATIONS

- Dose modifications may be necessary if urine creatinine clearance is less than 60 cc/minute.
- Epinephrine, corticosteroids, and antihistamines have been employed to alleviate anaphylactic-like symptoms.

Selected Readings

Alberts DS, Canetta R, Mason-Liddil N. Carboplatin in the first-line chemotherapy of ovarian cancer. *Semin Oncol.* 1990;**17(1)**:54-60.

Canetta R, Rozencweig M, Carter SK. Carboplatin: The clinical spectrum to date. *Cancer Treat Rev.* 1985;**12**(supple A):125-136.

Motzer RJ, Bosl GJ, Taver K, et al. Phase II trial of carboplatin in patients with advanced germ cell tumors refractory to cisplatin. *Cancer Treat Rep.* 1987;**71**:197-198.

Carmustine

BiCNU®, BCNU

MECHANISM OF ACTION

A nitrosourea, carmustine acts primarily as an alkylating agent. It interferes with DNA and RNA synthesis through alkylation.

METABOLISM/EXCRETION

Rapidly degraded with no intact drug detectable after 15 minutes when given intravenously. Antineoplastic and toxic effects may be due to its metabolites. 60%-70% of the dose is excreted in the urine after 96 hours and about 10% is excreted as respiratory CO_2. Highly lipid soluble; crosses the blood brain barrier.

INDICATIONS

1. Brain tumors*: glioblastoma, brainstem glioma,

medulloblastoma, astrocytoma, ependymoma,
metastatic brain tumors
2. Multiple myeloma*
3. Hodgkin's disease*
4. Non-Hodgkin's lymphomas*
5. Malignant melanoma

DOSAGE AND SCHEDULE
Adult
The recommended dose of BiCNU as a single agent in
previously untreated patients is 150-200 mg/m^2 IV every
6 weeks. This may be given as a single dose or divided
doses into daily injections such as 75-100 mg/m^2 on 2
successive days. When BiCNU is used in combination
with other myelosuppressive drugs or in patients in
whom bone marrow is depleted, the doses should be
adjusted accordingly. Doses subsequent to the initial
dose should be adjusted according to the hematologic
response of the patient to the preceding dose. (See
manufacturer's guide-line for dosage adjustments based
on nadir blood counts).

**A repeat course of BiCNU should not be given
until circulating blood elements have returned to
acceptable levels (platelets above 100,000/mm^3;
leukocytes above 4,000/mm^3); this usually occurs in 6
weeks.** Adequate number of neutrophils should be
present on a peripheral blood smear. Blood counts
should be monitored weekly and repeat courses should
not be given before 6 weeks because the hematologic
toxicity is delayed and cumulative.

Pediatric
Safety and effectiveness in children have not been
established.

ADMINISTRATION
Intravenous: Carmustine is given IV drip over 1-2
hours. Faster administration is associated with intense
pain and burning at the injection site.

STABILITY
Each package supplied contains 100 mg carmustine and a
vial of 3 ml sterile diluent. After reconstitution, BCNU
is stable for 8 hours at room temperature (25°C) or 24
hours under refrigeration (4°C).

DRUG INTERACTIONS

- Cimetidine (H$_2$ antagonist) may increase the toxic effects of carmustine.
- Amphotericin may enhance the cellular uptake of carmustine.

SIDE EFFECTS AND TOXICITIES

Hematologic

Delayed and cumulative myelosuppression is the dose-limiting toxicity occurring 4-6 weeks after treatment; thrombocytopenia nadir occurs in 4 weeks and lasts 1-2 weeks; leukopenia nadir occurs in 5-6 weeks and lasts 1-2 weeks after carmustine; anemia.

Gastrointestinal

Nausea and vomiting may occur 2 hours after a dose and can last 4-6 hours and may be dose-related; anorexia, diarrhea, stomatitis; hepatic toxicity (reversible): increased SGOT, alkaline phosphatase, bilirubin.

Renal

Nephrotoxicity (progressive azotemia, decrease in kidney size, renal failure); renal failure may be fatal.

Pulmonary

Pulmonary fibrosis may present with an insidious cough, dyspnea, or a sudden onset of respiratory failure; pulmonary fibrosis and/or pulmonary infiltrates have occurred 9 days to 43 months after treatment in patients receiving *cumulative doses* greater than 1400 mg/m^2, but can occur at lower doses; other risk factors include past history of lung disease and duration of treatment; pulmonary fibrosis (delayed onset) has occurred up to 15 years later in children and early adolescent patients treated with carmustine (cumulative doses 770-1800 mg/m^2) and cranial irradiation; pulmonary fibrosis may be progressive and fatal.

Dermatologic

Pain and/or burning may occur at the IV site or in the extremity during administration; facial flushing is more pronounced with faster administration rates; skin contact with carmustine may cause brown staining and pain.

Hypersensitivities

Contraindicated in patients with a previous hypersensitivity; as with all drugs, hypersensitivity, allergic reactions, and anaphylaxis may occur.

Reproductive

The drug is mutagenic and teratogenic.

Secondary Neoplasias

Acute leukemia and bone marrow dysplasia with long-term nitrosourea use.

Miscellaneous

Optic neuroretinitis and gynecomastia.

WARNINGS/PRECAUTIONS

- Hematologic monitoring is required during treatment and for at least 6 weeks after dosage.
- Pulmonary toxicity appears to be dose-related. Patients receiving greater than 1400 mg/m^2 are at higher risk of developing pulmonary toxicity.
- Pregnancy category D. It is not known if carmustine is excreted in human milk.

SPECIAL CONSIDERATIONS

- Strategies to decrease pain and/or burning during administration include further diluting carmustine, slowing the administration rate of carmustine, increasing the rate of the primary intravenous infusion, and/or placing ice above IV site.
- Pulmonary function tests should be obtained at baseline and repeated during treatment. Patients with a baseline below 70% of the predicted Forced Vital Capacity or Carbon Monoxide Diffusing Capacity are at risk of developing pulmonary toxicity.

Selected Readings

Anderson T, DeVita VT, Young RC. BCNU (NSC-409963) in the treatment of advanced Hodgkin's disease: Its role in remission introduction and maintenance. *Cancer Treat Rep.* 1976;**60**(6):761-767.

Holoye PY, Jenkins DE, Greenberg SD. Pulmonary toxicity in long-term administration of BCNU. *Cancer Treat Rep.* 1976;**60**:1691-1693.

Lokich JJ, Drum DW, Kaplan W. Hepatic toxicity of nitrosourea analogues. *Clin Pharmacol Ther.* 1974;**16**:363-367.

Oliverio VT. Toxicology and pharmacology of the nitrosoureas. *Cancer Chemother Rep Part 3.* 1973;**4**:13-20.

Chlorambucil

Leukeran®
MECHANISM OF ACTION
An alkylating agent, chlorambucil has a primary effect on preformed DNA, causing breaks in DNA strands and cross-links in DNA, thus preventing DNA, RNA, and protein synthesis. Derivative of nitrogen mustard. Cell cycle nonspecific. Damage is inflicted on resting and dividing cells.
METABOLISM/EXCRETION
Chlorambucil is extensively metabolized in the liver and excreted in the urine (60% of the drug metabolites are eliminated within 24 hours). Half-life: 1.5-2.5 hours. Well-absorbed orally, with an absolute oral bioavailability of 75.5% if taken with food.
INDICATIONS
1. Chronic lymphocytic leukemia*
2. Hodgkin's* and non-Hodgkin's lymphoma*
3. Lymphosarcoma*
4. Giant follicular lymphoma*
5. Carcinoma of the ovary and breast
6. Choriocarcinoma
DOSAGE AND SCHEDULE
Adult
The usual oral dosage is 0.1-0.2 mg/kg body weight daily for 3-6 weeks as required. This usually amounts to 4-10 mg/day for the average patient. The entire daily dose should be given at one time. These dosages are for the initiation of therapy or for short courses of treatment. The dosage must be carefully adjusted to the response of the patient and must be reduced as soon as there is an abrupt fall in the white blood cell count. Patients with Hodgkin's disease usually require 0.2 mg/kg/day, whereas patients with other lymphomas or chronic lymphocytic leukemia usually require only 0.1 mg/kg/day. When lymphocytic infiltration of the bone marrow is present, or when the bone marrow is hypoplastic, the daily dose should not exceed 0.1 mg/kg (about 6 mg for the average patient).

Alternate schedules for the treatment of chronic

lymphocytic leukemia employing intermittent, biweekly, or once-a-month pulse doses of chlorambucil have been reported. Intermittent schedules of chlorambucil begin with an initial single dose of 0.4 mg/kg. Doses are generally increased by 0.1 mg/kg until control of lymphocytosis or toxicity is observed. Subsequent doses are modified to produce mild hematologic toxicity. It is felt that the response rate of chronic lymphocytic leukemia to the biweekly or once monthly schedule of chlorambucil administration is similar or better than that previously reported with daily administration and that the hematologic toxicity was less than or equal to that encountered in studies using daily chlorambucil.

Radiation and cytotoxic drugs render the bone marrow more vulnerable to damage and chlorambucil should be used with particular caution within 4 weeks of a full course of radiation or chemotherapy. However, small doses of palliative radiation over isolated foci remote from the bone marrow will not usually depress the neutrophil and platelet count. In these cases chlorambucil may be given in the customary dosage.

It is presently felt that short courses of treatment are safer than continuous maintenance therapy although both methods have been effective. It must be recognized that continuous therapy may give the appearance of "maintenance" in patients who are actually in remission and have no immediate need for further treatment. If maintenance dosage is used, it should not exceed 0.1 mg/kg/day and well may be as low as 0.03 mg/kg/day. A typical maintenance dose is 2-4 mg/day, or less, depending on the status of the blood counts. It may, therefore, be desirable to withdraw the drug after maximal control has been achieved, since intermittent therapy reinstituted at the time of relapse may be as effective as continuous treatment.

Pediatric

The safety and effectiveness in children have not been well established.

ADMINISTRATION

Oral: 2 mg sugar-coated tablets.

STABILITY
Store at room temperature (15°-25°C or 59°-77°F).
DRUG INTERACTIONS
- Barbiturates may increase the toxicity of chlorambucil.
- There are no known drug-to-drug interactions with chlorambucil.

SIDE EFFECTS AND TOXICITIES
Hematologic
Myelosuppression, neutropenia, and thrombocytopenia may be dose-limiting and prolonged; leukopenia can be delayed up to 3 weeks and may continue for 10 days following the last dose of therapy, then rapidly return to normal; lymphocytopenia may occur with prolonged use; irreversible bone marrow damage has been reported.
Gastrointestinal
Nausea and vomiting (higher dosages); anorexia, weight loss, gastric distress, diarrhea, stomatitis, hepatotoxicity, jaundice hepatitis, abnormal liver function.
Renal
Hyperuricemia
Pulmonary
Pulmonary fibrosis, alveolar damage, and pneumonitis (rare), can be life-threatening
Neurologic
Seizures and coma (high-dose levels); myoclonic seizures have been described following an overdose of chlorambucil; seizures are more common in children treated with chlorambucil for nephrotic syndrome; severe periorbital edema, diplopia, and retinal hemorrhage; peripheral neuropathies, tremors, muscle twitching, confusion, agitation, ataxia, flaccid paresis, and hallucinations; drug fever
Dermatologic
Urticaria of the face and scalp, pustular eruption on mouth, chin, cheeks, and an urticarial erythema on the trunk that may spread to the legs; it usually occurs early in the treatment period and may last 10 days after the last dose; alopecia
Secondary Neoplasia
Acute myelogenous leukemia; mutagenic, teratogenic,

and carcinogenic properties.
Reproductive
Amenorrhea/azoospermia.
WARNINGS/PRECAUTIONS
- Pregnancy category D. It is not known whether the drug is excreted in human milk.
- Concomitant exposure to pneumococcus vaccination should be avoided.
- Contraindicated within 1 month of radiation or cytotoxic therapy; patients with thrombocytopenia, recent small pox vaccine, seizure history, or head trauma.

SPECIAL CONSIDERATIONS
- Concomitant use of allopurinol or colchicine may require dose reduction of these agents, because of chlorambucil-associated hyperuricemia.

Selected Readings

Byrne TN Jr, Moseley TAE III, Finer MA. Myoclonic seizures following chlorambucil overdose. *Ann Neurol.* 1981;**9**:191-194.

Knisley RE, Settipane GA, Albala MM. Unusual reaction to chlorambucil in a patient with chronic lymphocytic leukemia. *Arch Dermatol.* 1971;**104**:77-79.

Knopse WH, Loeb V Jr, Huguley CM Jr. Bi-weekly chlorambucil treatment of chronic lymphocytic leukemia. *Cancer.* 1974;**33**:555-561.

Millard LG, Rajah SM. Cutaneous reaction to chlorambucil. *Arch Dermatol.* 1977;**113**:1298.

Peterman A, Braunstein B. Cutaneous reaction to chlorambucil therapy. *Arch Dermatol.* 1986;**122**:1358-1360.

Williams SA, Makker SP, Grupe WE. Seizures—A significant side effect of chlorambucil therapy in children. *J Pediatr.* 1978;**93**:516-518.

Cisplatin

Platinol®, platinum, CDDP, DDP, Platinol®-AQ, CACP, cis-Diamminedichloroplatinum (II)

MECHANISM OF ACTION
A heavy metal platinum complex similar to bifunctional alkylating agents. The antitumor effect has been attributed to binding of DNA, production of interstrand

and intrastrand DNA cross-links, and formation of DNA adducts, thus preventing DNA, RNA, and protein synthesis. Cell cycle nonspecific.

METABOLISM/EXCRETION

Metabolism is not fully understood. Half-life: 73-290 hours. Twenty percent to 74% of the drug is excreted in the urine within 24-48 hours.

INDICATIONS

1. Carcinoma of the head and neck (squamous cell), testis*, ovary*, endometrial, cervical, bladder*, and gastrointestinal
2. Non-small cell and small cell lung cancer
3. Osteosarcoma and other soft-tissue sarcomas
4. Lymphoma
5. Pediatric brain tumors

DOSAGE AND SCHEDULE

Needles or intravenous sets containing aluminum parts that may come in contact with Platinol should not be used for preparation or administration. Aluminum reacts with Platinol, causing precipitate formation and a loss of potency.

Adult

Metastatic testicular tumors:

The usual Platinol dose for the treatment of testicular cancer in combination with other approved chemotherapeutic agents is 20 mg/m^2 IV daily for 5 days.

Metastatic ovarian tumors:

An effective combination for the treatment of patients with metastatic ovarian tumors includes Platinol and doxorubicin in the following doses: Platinol—50 mg/m^2 IV once every 3 weeks (day 1); doxorubicin—50 mg/m^2 IV once every 3 weeks (day 1). In combination therapy, Platinol and doxorubicin are administered sequentially. As a single agent, Platinol should be administered at a dose of 100 mg/m^2 IV once every 4 weeks.

Advanced bladder cancer:

Platinol should be administered as a single agent at a dose of 50-70 mg/m^2 IV once every 3-4 weeks depending on the extent of prior exposure to radiation therapy and/or prior chemotherapy. For heavily pretreated patients an initial dose of 50 mg/m^2 repeated every 4 weeks is recommended.

Pretreatment hydration with 1 to 2 l of fluid infused over 8-12 hours before a Platinol dose is recommended. Adequate hydration and urinary output must be maintained during the following 24 hours.

A repeat course of Platinol should not be given until the serum creatinine is below 1.5 mg/100 ml, and the BUN is below 25 mg/ml. A repeat course should not be given until circulating blood elements are at an acceptable level (platelets $\geq$ 100,000/mm^3, WBC $\geq$ 4,000/mm^3). Subsequent doses of Platinol should not be given until an audiometric analysis indicates that auditory acuity is within normal limits.

Pediatric
Safety and effectiveness have not been well established in children.

ADMINISTRATION
Intravenously, as *IV push, IV slow infusion,* or *continuous infusion* at a rate no greater than 1 mg/minute. The aqueous solution (Platinol-AQ) should be used intravenously only and should be administered by IV infusion over 6-8 hours. Avoid aluminum needles when administering, since a precipitate will form.

STABILITY
Available in 10 or 50 mg powder vials, or as an aqueous solution. Reconstituted solution is stable for 20 hours at room temperature. Do not place solution in the refrigerator or a precipitate will form. Protect diluted solution from light if it will not be used within 6 hours.

DRUG INTERACTIONS
- Ototoxicity increases when cisplatin is given with loop diuretics.
- Renal toxicity increases when cisplatin is given with aminoglycosides.
- Cisplatin decreases the effect of phenytoin; therefore, the dose of phenytoin may need to be increased.

SIDE EFFECTS AND TOXICITIES
Hematologic
Myelosuppression is dose-dependent; leukocyte nadir in

18-23 days with recovery in 39 days; anemia and
Coombs'-positive anemia.

Gastrointestinal

Acute and delayed nausea and vomiting occurs in the
majority of patients, usually severe, and can last up to 5
days; hepatic toxicity; persistent anorexia and taste
alterations.

Renal

Cumulative renal toxicity is severe; nephrotoxicity is
dose-dependent and dose-limiting occurring in 28%-
36% patients receiving moderate doses (50 mg/m²) and
manifested by renal tubular damage; the peak effect on
renal function usually occurs between 10 and 20 days
after therapy; renal damage is routinely reversible; the
renal protective effect of concomitant hydration and
mannitol diuresis is well documented; cisplatin also
causes potassium, calcium, phosphatase, and magnesium
wasting; hyperuricemia (SIADH) responsive to
allopurinol.

Pulmonary

Pulmonary fibrosis.

Cardiotoxic

Possible cardiotoxicity includes ST-T wave
abnormalities, bundle branch block, atrial fibrillation,
angina, myocardial infarction, and supraventricular
tachycardia.

Neurologic

Neuropathies (irreversible paresthesias) ("stocking-
glove" syndrome), loss of motor function, areflexia, and
loss of proprioception and vibratory sensation; focal
encephalopathy with associated cortical blindness,
seizures, and aphasia.

Dermatologic

Rare cellulitis and fibrosis of local tissue if extravasation
occurs.

Secondary Neoplasias

The drug has mutagenic and possibly teratogenic and
carcinogenic properties; acute leukemia coincident with
cisplatin is rare.

Hypersensitivities

Hypersensitivity reactions, manifested by anaphylaxis,

tachycardia, wheezing, flushing, facial edema, bronchoconstriction, and hypotension may occur within minutes of the infusion; treat with epinephrine, antihistamines, and corticosteriods, according to hospital policy and procedure, under the supervision of a physician.

Reproductive

Impotence, sterility, gynecomastia.

Miscellaneous

Cumulative ototoxicity is more pronounced in children and may be dose-related in all patients; ototoxicity is manifested by high frequency hearing loss above normal speech and occasional tinnitus; hearing loss may be unilateral or bilateral.

WARNINGS/PRECAUTIONS

- Contraindicated in patients with known hypersensitivity to platinum-containing compounds, impaired renal function, impaired hearing, myelosuppression, history of gout or renal stones, nursing and pregnant women (category D).
- Caution is advised when used in patients previously treated with radiation or cytotoxic agents, preexisting peripheral neuropathies, and with other ototoxic and nephrotoxic drugs.

SPECIAL CONSIDERATIONS

- Vigorous hydration before and after administration of cisplatin is recommended.
- Maintain urine output at least 100-150 ml/hour. Mannitol or furosemide diuresis may be necessary to maintain this output volume, especially with high-dose therapy.
- Serum creatinine, BUN, urine creatinine clearance, magnesium, sodium, potassium, and calcium should be obtained before therapy and monitored intermittently between courses and especially before initiating each subsequent course.
- Increasing potassium and magnesium intake through intravenous supplements and/or diet may be necessary.

Selected Readings

Cox EB, Burton GV, Olsen GA, Vugrin D. Cisplatin and etoposide: An effective treatment for refractory breast carcinoma. *Am J Clin*

Oncol. 1989;**12**(1):53-56.

Hainsworth JD, Johnson DH, Hande KR, Greco FA. Chemotherapy of advanced non-small cell lung cancer: A randomized trial of three cisplatin-based chemotherapy regimens. *Am J Clin Oncol.* 1989;**12**(4):345-359.

Kovnar E, McHaney V, Ayers D, et al. Effects of treatment sequence on ototoxicity due to cisplatin and radiation in pediatric brain tumor patients. *Proc Am Soc Clin Oncol.* 1991;**10**:311.

Menard O, Martinet Y, Lamy P. Cisplatin-induced atrial fibrillation. *J Clin Oncol.* 1990;**8**:192-193.

Sexauer C, Khan A, Burger P, et al. Cisplatinum in recurrent pediatric brain tumors: A POG phase II study (abstract). *Proc Am Soc Clin Oncol.* 1984;**8**:84.

Von Hoff DD, Slavik M, Muggia FM. Allergic reactions to cis-platinum (letter). *Lancet.* 1976;**1**:90.

Cyclophosphamide

Cytoxan®, CTX, Neosar®, Endoxan®, Endoxana, CPM

MECHANISM OF ACTION

A cell cycle nonspecific alkylating agent. Cyclophosphamide is activated by hepatic microsomal enzymes and then interferes in the growth of rapidly proliferating malignant cells. The mechanism of action is thought to involve the cross-linking of DNA in tumor cells. Because the cell continues to synthesize RNA and protein, an imbalance occurs and the cell dies.

METABOLISM/EXCRETION

Metabolized in the liver. Eliminated primarily as metabolites, with 5%-25% of unchanged drug excreted in the urine. Half-life: 4-6.5 hours.

INDICATIONS

1. Malignant lymphomas*: Hodgkin's and non-Hodgkin's disease, mixed cell type lymphoma; histiocytic lymphoma; Burkitt's lymphoma
2. Multiple myeloma*
3. Leukemias: chronic lymphocytic leukemia*, chronic granulocytic leukemia (however, usually ineffective in acute blast crisis), acute myelogenous and monocytic leukemia*, acute lymphoblastic stem-cell leukemia* in children (when given in remission is effective in prolonging its duration)
4. Advanced mycosis fungoides*

5. Disseminated neuroblastoma* and Wilm's tumor of childhood
6. Adenocarcinoma of the ovary*
7. Retinoblastoma*
8. Carcinoma of the breast*, lung, ovary*, testis, and bladder
9. Bone and soft tissue sarcomas
10. Rhabodomyosarcoma

DOSAGE AND SCHEDULE
Adult and Pediatric

When used as the only oncolytic drug therapy, the initial course of Cytoxan for patients with no hematologic deficiency usually consists of 40-50 mg/kg given intravenously in divided doses over a period of 2-5 days. Other intravenous regimens include 10-15 mg/kg given every 7-10 days or 3-5 mg/kg twice weekly.

Oral Cytoxan dosing is usually in the range of 1-5 mg/kg/day for both initial and maintenance dosing.

Many other regimens of intravenous and oral Cytoxan have been reported. Dosages must be adjusted in accord with evidence of antitumor activity and/or leukopenia. The total leukocyte count is a good, objective guide for regulating dosage. Transient decreases in the total white blood cell count to 2000 cells/mm³ (following short courses) or more persistent reduction to 3000 cells/mm³ (with continuing therapy) are tolerated without serious risk of infection if there is no marked granulocytopenia.

Patients with compromised renal function may show some measurable changes in pharmacokinetic parameters of Cytoxan metabolism, but there is no consistent evidence indicating a need for Cytoxan dosage modification in patients with renal function impairment.

ADMINISTRATION

Cyclophosphamide can be administered *orally* or *intravenously.* The drug may be given as IV push (in specific concentrations only) or diluted with D_5W or normal saline and administered by rapid or slow IV infusion. The total oral dose may be given at once or in divided doses. Adequate hydration (before treatment and 72 hours after) is necessary for high-dose intravenous therapy to reduce the incidence of hemorrhagic cystitis.

STABILITY

Available in 25 and 50 mg tablets. Available for intravenous injection: 100 mg, 200 mg, 500 mg, 1 gm, 2 gm vials. Stable at room temperature for 24 hours or, if a preservative is present in the diluent, refrigerated for 6 days. Store diluted vials at refrigerated temperatures between 2°-30° C (36°-86° F).

DRUG INTERACTIONS

- Barbiturates and other drugs that stimulate liver metabolic enzymes may increase the rate of hepatic conversion of cyclophosphamide to its toxic metabolites.
- Succinylcholine metabolism is blocked by cyclophosphamide, therefore, the neuromuscular blocking activity is prolonged.
- Cyclophosphamide increases chloramphenicol half-life.
- Thiazide diuretics increase duration of leukopenia from cyclophosphamide.
- Cyclophosphamide increases the effect of anticoagulants.
- Cyclophosphamide decreases digoxin levels. It may be necessary to increase the digoxin dose.
- Cyclophosphamide may potentiate doxorubicin-induced cardiotoxicty.

SIDE EFFECTS AND TOXICITIES

Hematologic

Leukopenia is the dose-limiting toxicity; rapid nadir is in 8-14 days and recovery in 18-25 days; thrombocytopenia can occur at high doses.

Gastrointestinal

Nausea and vomiting are dose-related and usually begin 2-4 hours after dosing, peak in 12 hours, and persist up to 24 hours; anorexia, mild stomatitis, abdominal discomfort or pain, and diarrhea; hepatotoxicity.

Renal

Hemorrhagic or non-hemorrhagic cystitis, which can be severe and fatal; most often it is reversible with discontinuation of the drug. The onset may be delayed from 24 hours to several weeks after therapy. Fibrosis of the bladder, sometimes extensive, may develop with or without accompanying cystitis. Forced fluids increases urinary frequency and output, thereby reducing the amount of time the drug remains in the bladder. Hematuria usually resolves a few days after cyclophosphamide is stopped, but it may persist. Mesna or other uroprotectors should be considered for all patients receiving high-dose cyclophosphamide therapy; medical and/or surgical supportive therapy in rare cases may be necessary to treat protracted cases of severe hemorrhagic cystitis; in severe cases, cyclophosphamide should be discontinued. Prolonged therapy may cause bladder cancer. Hyponatremia, hyperkalemia, hyperuricemia, weight gain without edema or weight loss. Inappropriate antidiuretic syndrome (SIADH) is common following IV doses greater than 50 mg/kg and is a limitation to and a consequence of fluid loading. Allopurinol and other thiazide-type diuretics potentiate the side effects of cyclophosphamide.

Pulmonary

Pulmonary toxicity is rare, but if it occurs, it may be lethal and is usually characterized by pneumonitis and is similar to "busulfan lung"; usually associated with long-term and continuous low-dose therapy. Glucocorticosteroids may be beneficial in treating this syndrome.

Cardiac

Cardiac toxicity occurs with high doses of cyclophosphamide (120-270 mg/kg administered over a period of a few days). With high doses of cyclophosphamide, severe, and sometimes fatal, congestive heart failure has occurred within a few days after the first dose. Histopathology has revealed hemorrhagic myocarditis; pericarditis has been reported independent of any hemopericardium.

Dermatologic

Alopecia, hyperpigmentation of nails and skin, transverse ridging of the nails, phlebitis at the injection site, nonspecific dermatitis.

Secondary Neoplasias
Carcinogenesis, mutagenesis, impairment of fertility, secondary malignancies.

Hypersensitivity
Anaphylaxis has occurred in rare instances.

Reproductive
Oligospermia or azoospermia and some degree of testicular atrophy may occur; azoospermia may be temporary; amenorrhea associated with decreased estrogen and increased gonadotropin secretion develops in a significant portion of women and may last up to 1 year after therapy. Ovarian fibrosis occurs with apparently complete loss of germ cells after prolonged use in late pubescence. Cyclophosphamide can cause irreversible sterility in both sexes.

WARNINGS/PRECAUTIONS
- Cyclophosphamide is contraindicated in patients with severely depressed bone marrow function and serious infections, nursing mothers, patients receiving live virus vaccines, and childbearing men and women.
- Cyclophosphamide should not be administered to those patients with a known hypersensitivity reaction.
- Pregnancy category D. Cyclophosphamide is excreted in human breast milk.
- Caution should be used in patients with a history of radiation therapy.

SPECIAL CONSIDERATIONS
- Give cyclophosphamide doses in the morning.
- Maintain ample fluid intake.
- Have patient empty bladder frequently, especially at bedtime.
- Rapid infusion may result in dizziness, nasal stuffiness, rhinorrhea, or nasal congestion occurring immediately or shortly thereafter.

Selected Readings

DeFronzo RA, Braine H, Colvin OM, et al. Water intoxication in man after cyclophosphamide therapy. Time course and relation to drug activation. *Ann Intern Med.* 1973;**78**:861-869.

DeVita VT, Serpick AA, Carbone PP. Combination chemotherapy in the treatment of advanced Hodgkin's disease. *Ann Intern Med.* 1970;**73**(6):881-895.

Rodin AE, Haggard ME, Travis LB. Lung changes and chemotherapeutic agents in childhood: Report of a case associated with cyclophosphamide therapy. *Am J Dis Child.* 1970;**120**:337-340.

Topelow AA, Rothenberg SP, Cottrell TS. Interstitial pneumonia after prolonged treatment with cyclophosphamide. *Am Rev Respir Dis.* 1973;**108**:114-117.

Cytarabine

Cytosar-U®, Cadastre-U, Ara-C, cytosine arabinoside

MECHANISM OF ACTION

An antimetabolite that is cell cycle specific. Pyrimidine analog affecting rapidly dividing cells in the S phase. Inhibits cell development from G_1 to S phase.

METABOLISM/EXCRETION

Metabolized primarily in the liver with a half-life of 1-3 hours. Eighty percent to 90% of the drug is excreted in the urine in 24 hours; the remainder is excreted in the bile. Moderate amounts of the drug cross the blood brain barrier. Cytarabine has crossed the placental barrier.

INDICATIONS

1. Acute non-lymphocytic leukemia* in adults and children
2. Acute myelogenous leukemia*
3. Acute lymphocytic leukemia
4. Chronic myelocytic leukemia
5. Intrathecal use in prophylaxis and treatment of CNS leukemia

DOSAGE AND SCHEDULE

Adult

In the induction therapy of acute non-lymphocytic leukemia, the usual dose in combination therapy with other anticancer drugs is 100 mg/m²/day by continuous infusion (days 1-7) or 100 mg/m² IV every 12 hours (days 1-7).

The literature should be consulted for the current recommendations for use in acute lymphocytic leukemia. Doses of 4.5 gm/m² by IV infusion over 1 hour every 12 hours for 12 doses has caused an unacceptable increase in irreversible CNS toxicity and death. Single doses as high as 3 gm/m^2 have been administered by rapid intravenous infusion without apparent toxicity.

Intrathecal use in meningeal leukemia:

Cytarabine has been used intrathecally in acute leukemia in doses ranging from 5-75 mg/m^2. The frequency of administration varies from once a day for 4 days to once every 4 days. The most frequently used dose is 30 mg/m^2 every 4 days until cerebrospinal fluid findings are normal, followed by one additional treatment. The dosage schedule is usually governed by the type and severity of central nervous system manifestations and the response to previous therapy. *If used intrathecally, do not use a diluent containing benzyl alcohol.*

Pediatric

Usually the same dose as adults. Safety and use in infants is not established.

ADMINISTRATION

The schedule and method of administration varies with the program of therapy to be used. Cytarabine may be given by *intravenous infusion* or *bolus injection, subcutaneously,* or *intrathecally.*

Patients can tolerate higher total doses when they receive the drug by rapid intravenous injection as compared with slow infusion. This phenomenon is related to the drug's rapid inactivation and brief exposure of susceptible normal and neoplastic cells to significant levels after rapid injection.

STABILITY

Supplied in 100 mg, 500 mg, 1 gm, and 2 gm multidose glass vials. Reconstituted drug is stable at room temperature for 48 hours and for 7 days when refrigerated.

DRUG INTERACTIONS

- The drug is incompatible with cephalothin, fluorouracil, gentamicin, heparin, insulin, nafcillin, oxacillin, and penicillin G.
- Digoxin levels must be monitored very carefully if used concomitantly with cytarabine.

SIDE EFFECTS AND TOXICITIES
Hematologic
Myelosuppression is the dose-limiting side effect; after 5 continuous days of therapy, the WBC has a biphasic nadir; nadir begins in 7-9 days, rises in 12, and falls again reaching full nadir in 15-24 days, with recovery 10 days following; anemia with megaloblastic changes in the bone marrow is common; immunosuppression of primary and secondary antibodies may occur.

Gastrointestinal
Nausea and vomiting with increased incidence and severity if the drug is given in divided doses, IV push or rapid infusion; diarrhea, stomatitis (7-10 days after therapy), anorexia, GI hemorrhage; transient hepatic dysfunction; hepatic toxicity with associated cholestatic jaundice with high doses of cytarabine.

Renal
Urinary retention and renal failure; tumor lysis syndrome if the patient has a large tumor bulk; this can occur 1-5 days after the first cycle of therapy.

Pulmonary
Pneumonia and dyspnea.

Cardiotoxic
Chest pain and cardiopathy.

Neurologic
High cumulative dose can lead to permanent CNS damage; dizziness, lethargy, and somnolence can occur with too rapid an infusion; CNS toxicities are more common in the elderly, but are usually mild and reversible.

Dermatologic
Maculopapular rash, fever, myalgia, bone pain, chest pain, conjunctivitis, and malaise (classic cytarabine syndrome); freckling, cellulitis, thrombophlebitis, pain and inflammation at subcutaneous injection sites, and alopecia.

Secondary Neoplasias
The drug is mutagenic and teratogenic.

Hypersensitivities
Flu-like syndrome of fever, arthralgia, and rash on the palms, soles, neck, and chest; rash is often related to

concomitant use of allopurinol; the rash on the palms and soles may be followed by bulla formation, desquamation, and eventual healing.

Reproductive

Cytarabine is teratogenic.

Miscellaneous

Conjunctivitis is seen with high-dose therapy; hydrocortisone eye drops, 2 drops OU QID for 10 days may ameliorate or prevent keratitis; it is recommended to start the eye drops the evening before therapy begins.

WARNINGS/PRECAUTIONS

- Contraindicated in patients with known hypersensitivity to the drug, renal and liver compromise, gout, and myelosuppression.
- Pregnancy (category D). It is not known if cytarabine is excreted in human milk.

SPECIAL CONSIDERATIONS

- Treat thrombophlebitis with warm compresses.
- High-dose therapy should not be infused in less than 1 hour.

Selected Readings

Altman AJ, Dinndorf P, Quinn JJ. Acute pancreatitis in association with cytosine arabinoside therapy. *Cancer.* 1982;**49:**1384-1386.

Jehn U, Goldel N, Rienmuller R, et al. Non-cardiogenic pulmonary edema complicating intermediate and high-dose Ara C treatment for relapsed acute leukemia. *Med Oncol Tumor Pharmacother.* 1988;**5**(1):41-47.

Levine LE, Medenica MM, Lorinez AL, et al. Distinctive acral erythema occurring during therapy for severe myelogenous leukemia. *Arch Dermatol.* 1985;**121:**102-104.

Rubin EH, Anderson JW, Berg DT. Risk factors for high-dose cytarabine neurotoxicity: An analysis of a cancer and leukemia Group B trial in patients with acute leukemia. *Cancer.* 1977;**44:**1189-1193.

Vaickus L, Letendre L. Pericarditis induced by high-dose cytarabine therapy. *Arch Intern Med.* 1984;**144:**1868-1869.

Dacarbazine

DTIC-Dome®, DIC, Imidazole carboxamide, dimethyl-triazeno-imdazol-carboxamide

MECHANISM OF ACTION
Alkylating agent that is postulated to be cell cycle nonspecific. The compound causes breakage and cross-linking of DNA strands, thus inhibiting DNA and RNA synthesis.

METABOLISM/EXCRETION
Metabolized extensively in the liver with 35%-50% excreted renally in 6 hours. Biphasic half-life, initial 35 minutes and terminal 5 hours. Five percent of the drug is protein bound.

INDICATIONS
1. Malignant melanoma*
2. Soft tissue sarcomas
3. Hodgkin's lymphoma* (refractory)
4. Neuroblastoma

DOSAGE AND SCHEDULE
Adult
Malignant melanoma:
The recommended dose is 2-4.5 mg/kg/day for 10 days, repeated at 4-week intervals. An alternate recommended dosage is 250 mg/m^2/day IV for 5 days. Treatment may be repeated every 3 weeks.

Hodgkin's disease:
The recommended dose of DTIC-Dome in the treatment of Hodgkin's disease is 150 mg/m^2/day IV for 5 days, in combination with other effective drugs, repeated every 4 weeks. An alternate dosage regimen is 375 mg/m^2 IV on day 1, in combination with other effective drugs, repeated every 15 days.

Pediatric
Safety and effectiveness have not been well established in children.

ADMINISTRATION
Both *intravenous push and infusion* methods have been used to administer dacarbazine. Administration using an IV push method should be done through a running line of normal saline or D_5W, verifying venous patency

before, during, and after infusion. Infusions are usually given over 15-30 minutes in 250-500 ml of fluid. Extravasation is likely to result in pain but not necrosis. Protecting the solution from light usually reduces venous irritation and discomfort.

STABILITY

Available in vials of 100, 200, and 500 mg of lyophilized drug. Reconstituted solution is stable for 8 hours at room temperature and 72 hours when refrigerated (4°C). The solution should be pale yellow; a pale pink color indicates decomposition. Dacarbazine rapidly deactivates (50% in 4 hours) if not protected from light. In contrast, if protected from light for 24 hours, only 5% loss of activity is detected.

DRUG INTERACTIONS

- Incompatible with heparin, lidocaine, and hydrocortisone.
- Decreased effectiveness when given with phenytoin and phenobarbital.

SIDE EFFECTS AND TOXICITIES

Hematologic

Mild to moderate myelosuppression, leukopenia and thrombocytopenia nadir between 21 and 25 days; however, leukopenia and thrombocytopenia can cause death; anemia.

Gastrointestinal

Nausea and vomiting are severe with an onset in 1-3 hours and a duration period lasting up to 12 hours; the intensity and severity of nausea and vomiting decrease with each subsequent dosing; aggressive antiemetic therapy is advised; hepatic failure, acute dystrophy with fatal thrombosis, anorexia.

Cardiotoxic

Hypotension with high-dose therapy.

Neurologic

Confusion, headache, seizures, and blurred vision with high-dose therapy; facial flushing and facial paresthesia.

Dermatologic

Alopecia; drug is an irritant; erythematous and/or urticarial rash; high-dose therapy may result in severe sun reactions (e.g., intense burning and pain with sun exposure).

Secondary Neoplasias

Dacarbazine has carcinogenic, mutagenic, and teratogenic properties.

Hypersensitivities

Anaphylaxis has occurred.

Reproductive

Dacarbazine is teratogenic.

Miscellaneous

Flu-like syndrome with malaise, fever, hypotension, and myalgia with an onset of 7 days and lasting for 1-3 weeks.

WARNINGS/PRECAUTIONS

- Pregnancy category C. It is not known whether the drug is excreted in human milk.
- Contraindicated with concomitant use of radiation therapy.

SPECIAL CONSIDERATIONS

- Diluting the drug in 100-200 ml of D_5W, slowing the infusion time, and applying ice to the infusion site/arm may reduce the pain and discomfort associated with the administration of dacarbazine.
- Patients should be advised to avoid the sun and wear sun protection with an SPF greater than 15.

Selected Readings

Ceci G, Bella M, Melissari M, et al. Fatal hepatic vascular toxicity of DTIC. Is it really a rare event? *Cancer.* 1988;**61**:1988-1991.

Feaux de Lacroix W, Runne W, Hauk U, et al. Acute liver dystrophy with thrombosis of hepatic veins: A fatal complication of dacarbazine treatment. *Cancer Treat Rep.* 1983;**67**:779-784.

Frosch PJ, Czarnetzki BM, Macher E, et al. Hepatic failure in a patient treated with dacarbazine (DTIC) for malignant melanoma. *J Cancer Res Clin Oncol.* 1979;**95**:281-286.

Dactinomycin-D

Actinomycin-D, Act-D, Cosmegen®

MECHANISM OF ACTION

An antitumor antibiotic, dactinomycin-D intercalates between base pairs of DNA resulting in inhibition of

DNA replication and RNA and protein synthesis. Cell cycle nonspecific; also has activity in the G_1 phase.

METABOLISM/EXCRETION

Minimally metabolized. Greater distribution of drug is found in the bone marrow than plasma. The majority of the drug is excreted in the urine. Thirty percent of the drug is found in urine and feces after 1 week. Plasma half-life is 36-48 hours.

INDICATIONS

1. Wilms' tumor*
2. Rhabdomyosarcoma*
3. Carcinoma of the testis and uterus*
4. Ewing's sarcoma*
5. Gestational choriocarcinoma
6. Melanoma

DOSE AND SCHEDULE

Toxic reactions to dactinomycin are frequent and may be severe, thus limiting in many instances the amount that may be given. However, the severity of toxicity varies markedly and is only partly dependent on the dose employed. The drug must be given in short courses.

The intravenous dosage of dactinomycin varies depending on the tolerance of the patient, the size and location of the tumor, and the use of other forms of therapy. It may be necessary to decrease the usual dosages suggested below when other chemotherapy or x-ray therapy is used concomitantly or has been used previously.

Adult and Pediatric

The dosage for adults or children should not exceed 15 μg/kg or 400-600 μg/m² daily IV for 5 days. The greater frequency of toxic effects of dactinomycin in infants suggests that this drug should be given to infants over the age of 6-12 months. Calculation of the dosage for obese or edematous patients should be on the basis of surface area in an effort to relate dosage to lean body mass.

Adults:

The usual adult dosage is 500 μg (0.5 mg) daily IV for a maximum of 5 days.

Children:

In children 15 µg/kg (0.015 mg/kg) is given IV daily for 5 days. An alternate schedule is a total dosage of 2500 µg/m^2 (2.5 mg/m^2) given IV over a 1-week period.

In both adults and children, a second course may be given after at least 3 weeks have elapsed, provided all signs of toxicity have disappeared.

ADMINISTRATION

Intravenous: Infuse slowly into the tubing or sidearm of a freely running intravenous infusion of normal saline or D$_5$W. *Vesicant properties:* Severe local tissue necrosis will result if the drug is inadvertently administered into the subcutaneous tissue.

STABILITY

Available as a lyophilized powder in vials containing 500 µg (0.5 mg) of dactinomycin and 20 mg of mannitol. Any unused portion of reconstituted drug should be discarded after 24 hours.

DRUG INTERACTIONS

- Dactinomycin may interfere with the determination of antibacterial drug levels.
- Additive hepatotoxicity may result with general anesthesia.

SIDE EFFECTS/TOXICITIES

Hematologic

Myelosuppression is the dose-limiting toxicity, occurring 7-10 days after treatment with nadir 14-21 days, recovery in 21-28 days, affecting primarily the platelets and leukocytes; delayed anemia.

Gastrointestinal

Nausea and vomiting are severe, occur within 1-2 hours and last for 4-20 hours; mucositis can occur within 5-7 days; diarrhea and gastrointestinal ulceration, hepatic toxicity (liver function abnormalities, ascites, hepatomegaly, hepatitis and hepato-veno-occlusive disease).

Dermatologic

Alopecia, radiation recall reaction, acne, hyperpigmentation of the skin, and increased sensitivity to sunlight; extravasation causing severe local tissue necrosis.

Hypersensitivity
Anaphylaxis.
Reproductive
May be mutagenic; the effect of dactinomycin on fertility has not been fully evaluated.
Secondary Neoplasias
Secondary malignancies may occur after dactinomycin; long-term follow up is required.
Miscellaneous
Hypocalcemia can occur from inhibition of osteoclast growth; malaise, fatigue, lethargy, fever, myalgia.
WARNINGS/PRECAUTIONS
- The dose of dactinomycin may need to be reduced when given in conjunction with radiation therapy or other chemotherapeutic agents, or if the patient has been previously treated.
- The myelosuppressive and gastrointestinal toxicity of dactinomycin may be increased when used in combination with radiation therapy.
- The administration of dactinomycin at or about the time of chicken pox or herpes zoster infection is contraindicated. A generalized disease resulting in death may occur.
- Contraindicated in patients who have had hypersensitivity or anaphylactic reactions to dactinomycin.
- Pregnancy (category C). A potential exists that dactinomycin is excreted in human milk.

SPECIAL CONSIDERATIONS
- Vesicant properties: severe tissue necrosis can result if dactinomycin is extravasated during administration.
- Patients should be advised to avoid the sun and wear sun protection with an SPF greater than 15.

Selected Readings

Frei E III. The clinical use of actinomycin. *Cancer Chemother Rep.* 1974;**58**:49-54.

Green DM, Norkool P, Breslow NE, et al. Severe hepatic toxicity after treatment with vincristine and dactinomycin using single-dose or divided-dose schedules: A report from the National Wilms' Tumor Study. *J Clin Oncol.* 1990;**8**:1525-1530.

Green DM, Sallan SE, Krishan A. Actinomycin D in childhood acute lymphoctic leukemia. *Cancer Treat Rep.* 1978;**62**:829-831.

Daunorubicin HCl

Daunomycin HCl, Cerubidine®

MECHANISM OF ACTION
Anthracycline antibiotic, daunorubicin HCl binds to nucleic acids by intercalation between the base pairs of DNA interfering with DNA synthesis. Causes inhibition of DNA topoisomerase II.

METABOLISM/EXCRETION
Binds extensively to tissue. Plasma half-life is 18.5 hours. Excreted primarily through the hepatobiliary route; about 40% of the drug is found in the bile. Urinary excretion accounts for approximately 25% of the dose.

INDICATIONS
1. Acute non-lymphocytic leukemia (myelogenous, monocytic, erythroid) remission induction in adults*
2. Acute lymphocytic leukemia (remission induction in adults and children)*

DOSAGE/SCHEDULE
To eradicate the leukemic cells and induce a complete remission, a profound suppression of the bone marrow is usually required. Evaluation of both the peripheral blood and bone marrow is mandatory in the formulation of appropriate treatment plans. It is recommended that the dosage of Cerubidine be reduced in instances of hepatic or renal impairment. See manufacturer guidelines for dose modifications based on serum bilirubin and serum creatinine.

DOSE SCHEDULES AND COMBINATION FOR THE APPROVED INDICATION OF REMISSION INDUCTION IN ADULT ACUTE NONLYMPHOCYTIC LEUKEMIA: For patients under age 60, Cerubidine 45 mg/m²/day IV on days 1,2,3 of the first course and on days 1,2 of subsequent courses AND cytosine arabinoside 100 mg/m²/day IV infusion daily for 7 days for the first course and for 5 days for subsequent courses.

For patients 60 years of age and above, Cerubidine 30 mg/m²/day IV on days 1,2,3 of the first course and on days 1,2 of subsequent courses AND cytosine arabinoside 100 mg/m²/day IV infusion daily for 7 days for the first course and for 5 days for subsequent courses. This Cerubidine dose reduction is based on a single study and may not be appropriate if optimal supportive care is available.

The attainment of a normal appearing bone marrow may require up to three courses of induction therapy. Evaluation of bone marrow following recovery from the previous course of induction therapy determines whether a further course of treatment is required.

DOSE SCHEDULE AND COMBINATION FOR THE APPROVED INDICATION OF REMISSION INDUCTION IN ADULT ACUTE LYMPHOCYTIC LEUKEMIA: IN COMBINATION—Cerubidine 45 mg/m²/day on days 1,2,3 AND vincristine 2 mg IV on days 1,8,15; prednisone 40 mg/m²/day PO on days 1-22, then tapered between days 22-29; L-asparaginase 500 IU/kg/day x 10 days IV on days 22-32.

DOSE SCHEDULE AND COMBINATION FOR THE APPROVED INDICATION OF REMISSION INDUCTION IN PEDIATRIC ACUTE LYMPHOCYTIC LEUKEMIA: IN COMBINATION—Cerubidine 25 mg/m²/day IV on day 1 every week, vincristine 1.5 mg/m² IV on day 1 every week, prednisone 40 mg/m² PO daily. Generally, a complete remission will be obtained within 4 such courses of therapy; however, if after 4 courses the patient is in partial remission, an additional 1 or, if necessary, 2 courses may be given in an effort to obtain a complete remission. In children < 2 years old or below 0.5 m² of body-surface area, it is recommended that the Cerubidine dosage calculation be based on weight (1 mg/kg) instead of body surface area.

ADMINISTRATION

Intravenous: The drug is injected into the sidearm of a rapidly flowing IV infusion of D_5W or normal saline. *Vesicant properties.*

STABILITY

Available in vials containing 20 mg of daunorubicin and 100 mg mannitol. Reconstituted solution is stable for 24

hours at room temperature and 48 hours refrigerated.
Protect from light.

DRUG INTERACTIONS
- Daunorubicin HCl may interact with a number of
  other drugs.

SIDE EFFECTS/TOXICITIES

Hematologic
Bone marrow suppression (dose-limiting toxicity); white
blood cell and platelet nadir 10-14 days.

Gastrointestinal
Nausea and vomiting, mild to moderate occurring 1-2
hours after treatment; diarrhea, mucositis (5-7 days after
treatment).

Renal
Urine may be red in color lasting 1-2 days;
hyperuricemia, renal and hepatic dysfunction (evidenced
by ↑bilirubin, ↑SGOT, ↑alkaline phosphatase).

Cardiac
Cardiotoxicity, acute and chronic (dose-limiting),
manifested by fatigue, dyspnea on exertion, and
arrhythmias; EKG changes during and after drug
administration; arrhythmias may be life-threatening;
delayed cardiomyopathy is dose-related presenting
symptoms similar to congestive heart failure (CHF),
which may be irreversible; pericarditis and myocarditis
have occurred; cardiotoxicity may take months to years
to present itself.

Dermatologic
Alopecia, anthracycline flare reaction, tissue necrosis if
extravasated, increased sensitivity to sunlight, facial
flushing, radiation recall reaction, hyperpigmentation of
the nail beds.

Hypersensitivities
As with all drugs, hypersensitive/allergic reactions and
anaphylaxis may occur.

Reproductive
The effect of daunorubicin on fertility has not been fully
evaluated.

Secondary Neoplasias
The drug may have carcinogenic and teratogenic
properties.

Miscellaneous
Fever, chills, rash (rare).
WARNINGS/PRECAUTIONS
- Increased toxicity to daunorubicin HCl may occur in patients with impaired hepatic or renal function. Dose reductions are recommended.
- EKG changes and a decrease in the systolic ejection fraction from baseline may be indicative of impending cardiotoxicity. Careful cardiac monitoring is required with EKGs and radionuclide angiography (RNCA) or echocardiography before, during, and after treatment with daunorubicin HCl. If test results indicate a change in cardiac function, the risk of continuing treatment must be carefully considered against the risk of developing irreversible cardiac damage.
- Preexisting cardiac disease and previous exposure to other anthracycline antibiotics or other cardiotoxic agents can increase the risk of cardiac toxicity. The total cumulative dose of daunorubicin HCl should take these conditions into account.
- Infants and children may be at greater risk of developing anthracycline-induced cardiotoxicity. Impaired left ventricular systolic function, reduced contractility, CHF, and death have been associated with anthracycline therapy in pediatric patients.
- Cumulative lifetime doses of daunorubicin HCl: Adults: < 550 mg/m^2 (higher doses increase risk of cardiotoxicity), < 400 mg/m^2 in patients with prior mediastinal radiation. Children: > 2 years old: 300 mg/m^2, < 2 years old: 10 mg/kg.
- Pregnancy category D. It is not known if the drug is excreted in human milk.

SPECIAL CONSIDERATIONS
- During administration of daunorubicin HCl, patients should be asked to report any signs of pain or burning or any other symptoms. Extravasation can occur in the presence of a good blood return and no complaints of pain and burning. Assessment of venous patency is required before, during, and after administration of doxorubicin. In the event of extravasation, early intervention is required. The area should be examined

frequently and a plastic surgeon consult should be considered.

- Patients should be advised to avoid the sun and wear sun protection with an SPF greater than 15.

Selected Readings

Gilladoga AC, Manuel C, Tan CTC, et al. The cardiotoxicity of Adriamycin and daunomycin in children. *Cancer.* 1976;**37**(suppl):1070-1078.

Jones B, Holland JF, Morrison AR, et al. Daunorubicin (NSC-82151) in the treatment of advanced childhood lymphoblastic leukemia. *Cancer Res.* 1971;**31**:84-90.

Lipshultz SE, Colan SD, Gelber RD, et al. Late cardiac effects of doxorubicin therapy for acute lymphoblastic leukemia in childhood. *N Engl J Med.* 1991;**324**:808-815.

Reaman GH, Ladisch S, Echelberger C, et al. Improved treatment results in the management of single and multiple relapses of acute lymphoblastic leukemia. *Cancer.* 1980;**45**:3090-3094.

Von Hoff DD, Rozencweig M, Layard M, et al. Daunomycin-induced cardiotoxicity in children and adults. *Am J Med.* 1977;**62**:200-208.

Yates J, Glidewell O, Wiernik P, et al. Cytosine arabinoside with daunorubicin or Adriamycin for therapy of acute myelocytic leukemia: A CALGB study. *Blood.* 1982;**60**(2):454-462.

Doxorubicin HCl

Adriamycin®, doxorubicin HCl, Adria, DOX

MECHANISM OF ACTION

An anthracycline antibiotic, doxorubicin binds to nucleic acids by intercalation with the base pairs of the DNA double helix interfering with DNA synthesis. Causes inhibition of DNA topoisomerase I and II.

METABOLISM/EXCRETION

Doxorubicin is rapidly distributed in body tissues, binding to plasma proteins and cell membranes. Excreted primarily through the hepatobiliary route; about 40%-50% of the drug is found in the bile and feces in 7 days. Urinary excretion accounts for approximately 4%-5% of the dose in 5 days.

INDICATIONS

1. Acute lymphoblastic leukemia*
2. Acute, myeloblastic leukemia*
3. Wilms' tumor*

4. Neuroblastoma*
5. Soft tissue and bone sarcomas*
6. Breast carcinoma*
7. Ovarian carcinoma*
8. Transitional cell bladder carcinoma*
9. Thyroid carcinoma*
10. Hodgkin's and non-Hodgkin's lymphoma*
11. Bronchogenic carcinoma (small cell type)*
12. Gastric carcinoma*

DOSAGE AND SCHEDULE
Adult
The most common used dosage schedule is 60-75 mg/m2 as a single IV injection administered at 21-day intervals. The lower dose should be given to patients with inadequate marrow reserve caused by old age, prior therapy, or neoplastic marrow infiltration. An alternative dose schedule is weekly doses of 20 mg/m2, which has been reported to produce a lower incidence of congestive heart failure. 30 mg/m2 on each of 3 successive days, repeated every 4 weeks has also been used. Adriamycin dosage must be reduced if the bilirubin is elevated as follows: serum bilirubin 1.2-3.0 mg/dl—give $1/2$ normal dose; > 3 mg/dl—give $1/4$ normal dose.

Pediatric
The safety and effectiveness have not been well established in children.

ADMINISTRATION
Intravenous: Infuse slowly into the tubing of a freely running intravenous infusion of normal saline or D_5W. Use a large vein. Rate of administration is dependent on the dose and size of vein. Administration rate should not be less than 3-5 minutes.

   VESICANT PROPERTIES. Severe local tissue necrosis can result if extravasation occurs during administration.

STABILITY
Reconstituted solutions should be protected from light if not used within 8 hours.

DRUG INTERACTIONS
• Doxorubicin may increase the incidence of cytoxan-

induced hemorrhagic cystitis.
- Hepatotoxicity associated with 6-mercaptopurine may be increased.

SIDE EFFECTS/TOXICITIES

Hematologic
Bone marrow suppression is one of the dose-limiting toxicities of doxorubicin; the white blood cell nadir can occur at 10-14 days and recover by day 21; the effect of doxorubicin on the platelets and RBCs is not as significant.

Gastrointestinal
Nausea and vomiting 1-2 hours after administration, the severity is dose-dependent; mucositis 5-7 days after treatment; anorexia, diarrhea, ulceration, and necrosis of the colon.

Renal
Red-colored urine may last 1-2 days; hyperuricemia.

Cardiac
Cardiotoxicity, acute and chronic, (dose-limiting); EKG changes have occurred during and after doxorubicin administration; arrhythmias may be life-threatening; delayed cardiomyopathy is dose-related presenting symptoms similar to congestive heart failure (CHF), which may be irreversible; cardiotoxicity may take months to years to occur.

Dermatologic
Alopecia, anthracycline flare reaction, tissue necrosis if extravasated, increased sensitivity to sunlight, facial flushing, radiation recall reaction, hyperpigmentation of the skin and nail beds.

Hypersensitivities
Fever, chills, and urticaria; anaphylaxis.

Reproductive
The potential adverse effect of doxorubicin on fertility is not known.

Secondary Neoplasias
May be carcinogenic, teratogenic, and mutagenic.

Miscellaneous
Conjunctivitis and excessive lacrimation have been reported.

WARNINGS/PRECAUTIONS

- An increase in the toxic effects of doxorubicin can occur in patients with impaired hepatic function. Dose reductions are recommended (see manufacturer's guidelines).
- Dose-related cardiac toxic effects can occur with doxorubicin. Maximum lifetime doses of doxorubicin are recommended, although the cardiotoxicity can occur at lower doses. The doses are: 550 mg/m^2 for the cumulative lifetime dose and 400 mg/m^2 in patients who have received prior mediastinal radiation or who have received concomitant therapy that is cardiotoxic.
- Careful cardiac monitoring is required with EKGs and radionuclide angiography (RNCA) or echocardiography before, during, and after treatment with doxorubicin. If test results indicate a change in cardiac function, the risk of continuing treatment must be carefully considered against the risk of developing irreversible cardiac damage.
- Doxorubicin is contraindicated in patients who have received previous treatment at cumulative doses of daunomycin or doxorubicin. The total doxorubicin dose must take these agents into account.
- Doxorubicin is contraindicated in patients with severe myelosuppression occurring from other treatment (chemotherapy or radiation therapy).
- Obesity can result in reduced clearance and increased toxicity.
- Pregnancy category D. It is not known if the drug is excreted in human milk.

SPECIAL CONSIDERATIONS

- During administration of doxorubicin, patients should be asked to report any signs of pain or burning or any other symptoms. Extravasation can occur in the presence of a good blood return and no complaints of pain and burning. Assessment of venous patency is required before, during, and after administration of doxorubicin. In the event of extravasation, early intervention is required. The area should be examined frequently and a plastic surgeon consult should be considered.

- Patients should be advised to avoid the sun and wear sun protection with an SPF greater than 15.

Selected Readings

Hryniuk W, Levine MN. Analysis of dose-intensity for adjuvant chemotherapy trials in stage II breast cancer. *J Clin Oncol.* 1986;**4:**1162-1170.

Lipshultz SE, Colan SD, Gelber RD, et al. Late cardiac effects of doxorubicin therapy for acute lymphoblastic leukemia in childhood. *N Engl J Med.* 1991;**324:**808-815.

Mattsson W, Borgstrom S, Landberg T, Trope C. A weekly schedule of low-dose doxorubicin in the treatment of advanced breast cancer. *Clin Ther.* 1982;**5**(2):193-203.

Minow RA, Benjamin RS, Gottlieb JA. Adriamycin (NSC-123127) cardiomyopathy—an overview with determination of risk factors. *Cancer Chemother Rep Part 3.* 1975;**66**(2):195-201.

Rudolph R, Stein R, Patillo RA. Skin ulcers due to adriamycin. *Cancer.* 1976;**38:**1087-1094.

Steinherz L, Steinherz P, Tan C, Murphy L. Cardiac toxicity 4-20 years after completing anthracycline therapy. *Proc Amer Soc Clin Oncol.* 1989;**8:**296.

Torti F, Bristow M, et al. Reduced cardiotoxicity of doxorubicin on a weekly schedule. *Ann Intern Med.* 1983;**99**(6):745-749.

Von Hoff DD, Layard MW, Basa P, et al. Risk factors for doxorubicin-induced congestive heart failure. *Ann Intern Med.* 1979;**91:**710-717.

Etoposide

VP-16, VePesid®

MECHANISM OF ACTION

A semisynthetic derivative of the podophyllotoxins. Etoposide inhibits DNA topoisomerase II, thereby inhibiting DNA synthesis. Cell cycle specific; active in the G_2 phase and to a lesser extent in the S phase. It does not interfere with microtubular assembly.

METABOLISM/EXCRETION

Majority of the drug is excreted in the urine (30%). Biliary excretion accounts for approximately 6% of the drug. Metabolism accounts for most of the nonrenal clearance of the drug. The initial half-life is 1.5 hours and the terminal elimination half-life range is 4-11 hours. Bioavailability of the oral capsules is approximately 50%

(range 25%-75%). Food and other chemotherapeutic agents do not affect the absorption of etoposide. There does not appear to be a difference in metabolism and excretion between the intravenous and oral forms.

INDICATIONS

1. Refractory testicular tumors*
2. Small cell lung cancer*
3. Relapsed Hodgkin's and non-Hodgkin's lymphoma
4. Acute non-lymphocytic leukemia
5. Gestational trophoblastic tumors
6. Ewing's sarcoma

DOSAGE AND SCHEDULE

Adult

VePesid for injection:

The usual dose of VePesid in testicular cancer in combination with other approved chemotherapeutic agents ranges from 50-100 mg/m^2/day on days 1-5 to 100 mg/m^2/day on days 1,3, and 5.

In small-cell lung cancer, the VePesid dose in combination with other approved chemotherapeutic drugs ranges from 35 mg/m^2/day for 4 days to 50 mg/m^2/day for 5 days.

Chemotherapy courses are repeated at 3- to 4-week intervals after adequate recovery from any toxicity.

VePesid capsules:

In small-cell lung cancer, the recommended dose of VePesid capsules is 2 times the IV dose rounded to the nearest 50 mg.

The dosage, by either route, should be modified to take into account the myelosuppressive effects of other drugs in the combination or the effects of prior x-ray therapy or chemotherapy, which may have compromised bone marrow reserve.

Pediatric

Safety and effectiveness in children have not been established. VePesid contains polysorbate 80.

ADMINISTRATION

Intravenous, IV piggyback over 30-60 minutes.
Irritant properties. Oral, capsules may be taken at the same time; no need to divide the dose.

STABILITY
VP-16 is available in multidose vials containing 100 mg/5ml, 150 mg/7.5ml, 500 mg/25 ml, and 1 gm/50ml. Oral VP-16 are available in 50 mg pink capsules. Reconstituted solutions of VP-16 are stable at concentrations of 0.4 mg/ml for 24 hours and concentration of 0.2 mg/ml for 96 hours at room temperature. Capsules of VP-16 must be refrigerated and are stable for 24 months.

DRUG INTERACTIONS
• Prior or concomitant treatment with other drugs that are renally excreted may decrease the clearance of etoposide, resulting in increased exposure. These can include but are not limited to, cisplatin, ifosfamide, and cyclosporin A.

SIDE EFFECTS AND TOXICITIES
Hematologic
Myelosuppression (dose limiting); granulocyte nadir 7-14 days after treatment; platelet nadir 9-16 days, recovery by day 20.

Gastrointestinal
Nausea and vomiting mild to moderate; mucositis (dose-limiting toxicity), anorexia, diarrhea, constipation, and abdominal pain; a metallic taste during administration; at higher doses hepatic toxicity and metabolic acidosis.

Pulmonary
Bronchospasm with severe wheezing during administration, usually responsive to antihistamines and corticosteroids.

Cardiac
Myocardial infarction and congestive heart failure in patients with preexisting heart disease.

Neurologic
Peripheral neuropathy (rare); preexisting peripheral neuropathy caused by vincristine may be exacerbated; somnolence and fatigue.

Dermatologic
Alopecia, rash, pruritus and/or urticaria, radiation recall reaction, Stevens-Johnson syndrome, facial flushing.

Hypersensitivities

Anaphylactic reactions in patients receiving intravenous etoposide and oral etoposide (rare); symptoms: fever, chills, tachycardia, bronchospasm, dyspnea, and/or hypotension; facial/tongue swelling, coughing diaphoresis, cyanosis, tightness in the throat, laryngospasm, back pain, and/or loss of consciousness; hypotension if infused too rapidly.

Reproductive

Potentially mutagenic and genotoxic.

Secondary Neoplasia

Potential carcinogen in humans.

Miscellaneous

Fever.

WARNINGS/PRECAUTIONS

- Etoposide contains polysorbate 80, which has been linked to liver and renal failure, pulmonary deterioration, thrombocytopenia, and ascites in premature infants.
- The use of etoposide is contraindicated in patients who have had a hypersensitivity or anaphylactic reaction to the drug.
- Dose reduction of etoposide is recommended for elevated bilirubin or for renal impairment. See manufacturer's guidelines.
- Elevated serum SGPT levels in children may result in decreased total body clearance of etoposide. An inverse relationship between plasma albumin levels and renal clearance is found in children. In adults the total body clearance is correlated with creatinine clearance, serum albumin, and nonrenal clearance.
- Pregnancy category D. Etoposide may be excreted in human milk.

SPECIAL CONSIDERATIONS

- Anaphylactic reactions are more common during the initial infusion of etoposide. Reactions can be fatal. Treatment consists of, but is not limited to, stopping the drug and administering antihistamines, corticosteroids, pressor agents, and/or volume expanders.
- Hypotension is usually rate-related. Etoposide should be administered slowly over a minimum of 30-60

minutes. In the event of hypotension, stop the drug immediately. Administer IV fluids or other supportive therapy as indicated. Slow the administration rate when restarting the infusion.

- Sucking on hard candy during drug administration may lessen the metallic taste.

Selected Readings

Aisner J, Whitacre M, VanEcho DA, et al. Doxorubicin cyclophosphamide and VP-16-213 (ACE) in the treatment of small-cell lung cancer. *Cancer Chemother Pharmacol.* 1982b;**7**:187-193.

Bosl GJ, Jain K, Dukeman M, et al. VP-16 and cisplatin (DDP) in the treatment of patients (PTS) with advanced germ cell tumors (GCT). *Proc Am Soc Clin Oncol.* 1982;**1**:114.

Einhorn LH, Penington K, McClean J. Phase II trial of daily oral VP-16 in refractory small-cell lung cancer: A Hoosier Oncology Group Study. *Semin Oncol.* 1990;**17**:32-35.

Joel S, Clark P, Slevin M. Renal function and etoposide pharmacokinetics: Is dose modification necessary? *Proc Am Soc Clin Oncol.* 1991;**10**:103.

Murphy SB. Secondary acute myeloid leukemia following treatment with epipodophyllotoxins (editorial). *J Clin Oncol.* 1993;**11**:199-201.

Perry MC. Hepatotoxicity of chemotherapeutic agents. *Semin Oncol.* 1982;**9**:65-74.

Slevin ML, Clark PI, Joel SP, et al. A randomized trial to evaluate the effect of schedule on the activity of etoposide in small-cell lung cancer. *J Clin Oncol.* 1989a;**7**:1333-1340.

Floxuridine

FUDR

MECHANISM OF ACTION

Pyrimidine antimetabolite that is cell cycle specific late in the S phase. Inhibits thymidylate synthesis, thus interfering with cell replication and inhibiting DNA synthesis.

METABOLISM/EXCRETION

Seventy percent to 90% of the drug is extracted by the liver in the first pass (this is a major advantage over 5-FU). Metabolites are excreted by the kidneys and lungs

(60%-80%). Biphasic half-life: initial 10-20 minutes, terminal at 20 hours. Crosses blood brain barrier.

INDICATIONS

1. Liver metastasis of GI adenocarcinomas*
2. Primary liver carcinomas
3. Oral cancers
4. Pancreatic carcinomas
5. Liver and biliary tract tumors
6. Adenocarcinoma of the breast

DOSAGE AND SCHEDULE

For intraarterial infusion only.

Adult

The recommended therapeutic dosage schedule of FUDR by continuous arterial infusion is 0.1-0.6 mg/kg/day. The higher dosage ranges (0.4-0.6 mg) are usually employed for hepatic artery infusion because the liver metabolizes the drug, thus reducing the potential for systemic toxicity. Therapy can be given until adverse reactions appear. When side effects have subsided, therapy may be resumed. The patient should be maintained on therapy as long as response to FUDR continues.

Pediatric

Safety and effectiveness in children have not been established.

ADMINISTRATION

Intraarterial (administration method of choice) via a surgically implanted catheter directed to the major artery supplying the well-defined tumor. FDA approval is for intrahepatic arterial infusion only. Administration is best achieved if used with an appropriate pump to assure uniform delivery and overcome pressure from large arteries. Intraarterial line is kept patent with a heparinized solution when the patient is not being treated.

STABILITY

Available in 500 mg/5 ml glass vial. Reconstituted solutions may be stored for 2 weeks if refrigerated.

DRUG INTERACTIONS

- Increased toxicity with concurrent radiation and antineoplastics.

SIDE EFFECTS AND TOXICITIES
Hematologic
Myelosuppression manifested by leukopenia and to a lesser degree thrombocytopenia; anemia

Gastrointestinal
Nausea and vomiting are mild and infrequent; diarrhea (mild to moderately severe), enteritis, stomatitis (early sign of severe toxicity), duodenal ulcer (10% occurrence), duodenitis, gastritis, bleeding, gastroenteritis, glossitis, pharyngitis, anorexia, abdominal pain and cramps, possible intra- and extra-hepatic biliary sclerosis, and acalculous cholecystitis; chemically induced hepatitis with elevated alkaline phosphatase.

Renal
Renal failure.

Cardiotoxic
Myocardial ischemia and angina.

Neurologic
Cerebellar ataxia, vertigo, nystagmus, seizures, depression, hemiplegia, hiccoughs, lethargy, and blurred vision may occur; CNS toxicities can be acute or delayed in occurrence.

Dermatologic
Localized erythema, alopecia, dermatitis, edema, hyperpigmentation of veins, and rash; "hand-foot syndrome" depicted by painful, erythematous desquamation and fissures of palms and soles; sun exposure tends to initiate and/or increase skin reactions.

Secondary Neoplasias
No evaluation on floxuridine's carcinogenic potential can be made based on available data.

Hypersensitivities
As with any drug, hypersensitive/allergic reactions and anaphylaxis are possible.

Reproductive
The drug has demonstrated mutagenic and teratogenic properties.

Miscellaneous
Procedural complications with the insertion of an arterial catheter and difficulties with regional arterial infusions (e.g., leakage, clots, catheter occlusions, dislodgement,

perforation, biliary sclerosis, and infections) are possible; fever, lethargy, weakness, and malaise.

WARNINGS/PRECAUTIONS

- Contraindicated in patients with poor nutritional status, depressed bone marrow function, and serious infections. Dose reduction is advised in these patients.
- Caution should be used in patients with impaired renal and/or hepatic function, a history of high-dose pelvic radiation, and previous treatment with alkylating agents.
- Pregnancy category D. It is not known if floxuridine is excreted in human milk.

SPECIAL CONSIDERATIONS

- When administered intraarterially, an H_2 antihistamine, ranitidine (150 mg PO BID), is recommended to prevent peptic ulcer disease while on therapy.

Selected Readings

Anderson N, Lokich J, Bern M, et al. Combined 5-fluorouracil and floxuridine administered as a 14-day infusion. A phase I study. *Cancer.* 1989;**63:**825-827.

Davis HL, Guillermo R, Ansfield FJ. Adenocarcinomas of stomach, pancreas, liver, and biliary tracts. *Cancer.* 1974;**33:**105-197.

Karnofsky DA, Young CW. Comparative aspects of the pharmacology of the antimetabolites. *Fed Proc.* 1967;**26:**1139-1145.

Kemeny N, Daly J, Reichman B, Geller N, et al. Intrahepatic or systemic infusion of fluorodeoxyuridine in patients with liver metastases from colorectal carcinoma. *Ann Intern Med. 1987;**107:**459-465.

Fludarabine phosphate

Fludara®, FLAMP

MECHANISM OF ACTION

An antimetabolite, fludarabine phosphate interferes with DNA synthesis by inhibiting ribonucleotide reductase.

METABOLISM/EXCRETION

Fludarabine phosphate is rapidly converted into an active metabolite (2 fluoro-ara-A or 2-FLAA) minutes after administration. Approximately 23% of the dose is excreted into the urine as 2-FLAA.

INDICATIONS

1. B-cell chronic lymphocytic leukemia (CLL)* that has not responded to or that has progressed during treatment with at least one standard alkylating chemotherapy regimen.
2. Low-grade lymphomas.
3. Mycosis fungoides.

DOSAGE AND SCHEDULE

Adult

The recommended dose of Fludara for Injection is 25 mg/m^2 IV over a period of approximately 30 minutes daily for 5 consecutive days. Each 5-day course of treatment should commence every 28 days. Dosage may be decreased or delayed based on evidence of hematologic or nonhematologic toxicity. Physicians should consider delaying or discontinuing the drug if neurotoxicity occurs. A number of clinical factors may predispose the patient to increased toxicity from Fludara. These factors include advanced age, renal insufficiency, and bone marrow impairment. Such patients should be monitored for excessive toxicity and the dose modified accordingly. The optimal duration of treatment has not been clearly established. It is recommended that 3 additional cycles of Fludara be administered following the achievement of a maximal response and then the drug should be discontinued.

Pediatric

Safety and effectiveness in children have not been established.

ADMINISTRATION

Intravenous: IV drip over 30 minutes.

STABILITY

Available in 50 mg vial. Reconstituted solutions do not contain preservatives. Unused solutions should be discarded after 8 hours.

DRUG INTERACTIONS

- The use of fludarabine phosphate in combination with pentostatin is not recommended because of the severe risk of pulmonary toxicity.

SIDE EFFECTS AND TOXICITIES
Hematologic
Myelosuppression (dose limiting and cumulative); nadir at 13 days with a range of 3-25 days; neutropenia, thrombocytopenia, and/or anemia; bone marrow fibrosis, and hemolytic anemia.
Gastrointestinal
Nausea, vomiting and diarrhea, anorexia, stomatitis; hepatic transaminase and serum creatine levels may increase; gastrointestinal bleeding.
Renal
Hyperuricemia, hyperphosphatemia, hematuria, urate crystalluria, renal failure, and hemorrhagic cystitis.
Pulmonary
Manifestations of pulmonary toxicity include dyspnea, cough, fever, hypoxia, interstitial pulmonary infiltrates, and effusions.
Cardiac
Edema and pericardial effusion.
Neurologic
Weakness, paresthesia, headache, agitation, confusion, visual disturbances, hearing loss, and coma; at doses higher than recommended for CLL ($25 \text{ mg/m}^2/\text{d} \times 5$ days), blindness, coma, and death have occurred.
Dermatologic
Skin rashes and pruritus.
Hypersensitivities
Contraindicated in patients with a prior hypersensitivity to the drug or its components.
Reproductive
The possible adverse effects on fertility have not been established.
Secondary Neoplasias
The drug may have carcinogenic properties.
Miscellaneous
Fatigue, myalgias, fever, and chills.
WARNINGS/PRECAUTIONS
- The safety and effectiveness of fludarabine phosphate in previously untreated or nonrefractory patients have not been established.
- Dose-dependent toxic effects can occur with

fludarabine phosphate. Severe neurologic effects have occurred at high doses of fludarabine phosphate, but it has rarely been reported at the recommended dose. The effect of long-term therapy on the CNS is not known.

- Use cautiously in patients with renal insufficiency.
- Pregnancy category D. It is not known if the drug is excreted in human milk.

SPECIAL CONSIDERATIONS

- Measures to prevent tumor lysis syndrome should be instituted before beginning treatment. Tumor lysis syndrome may include hyperuricemia, hyperphosphatemia, hypocalcemia, hyperkalemia, urate crystalluria, and renal failure. Symptoms may include flank pain and hematuria.

Selected Readings

Chun HG, Leyland-Jones BR, Caryk SM, Hoth DF. Central nervous system toxicity of fludarabine phosphate. *Cancer Treat Rep.* 1986;**70:**1225-1228.

Hurst PG, Habib MP, Garwal H, Bluestein M, Paguin M, Greenberg BR. Pulmonary toxicity associated with fludarabine monophosphate. *Invest New Drugs.* 1987;**5:**207-210.

Keating MJ, Kantarjian H, Talpaz M, et al. Fludarabine: A new agent with major activity against chronic lymphocytic leukemia. *Blood.* 1989;**74**(1):19-25.

Merkel DE, Griffin NL, Kagan-Hallat K, Von Hoff DD. Central nervous system toxicity with fludarabine. *Cancer Treat Rep.* 1986;**70:**1449-1450.

Warrell RP, Berman E. Phase I and II study of fludarabine phosphate in leukemia: Therapeutic efficacy with delayed central nervous system toxicity. *J Clin Oncol.* 1986;**4:**74-79.

5-Fluorouracil

5-FU, fluorouracil, Fluorouracil injection, Efudex®, Adrucil®, Fluoroplex®

MECHANISM OF ACTION

A cell cycle specific (S phase), "false" pyrimidine antimetabolite that inhibits the formation of the DNA-specific nucleoside base thymidine through inhibition of the thymidine synthetase and incorporation of FUTP into DNA and RNA.

METABOLISM / EXCRETION

Biphasic half-life: initial 8-20 minutes, terminal at 20 hours. Metabolized in the liver and excreted by the kidneys in the urine and by the lungs as carbon dioxide. Fluorouracil crosses the blood brain barrier and may cross the placental barrier.

INDICATIONS

1. GI malignancies: colon*, rectal*, stomach*
2. Breast*
3. Pancreas*
4. Head and neck cancer
5. Renal cell carcinoma
6. Squamous cell carcinoma of the esophagus
7. Prostate cancer
8. Topical use in basal cell carcinoma and a variety of other malignant dermatoses
9. Intraarterial use in liver cancer

DOSAGE AND SCHEDULE

All dosages should be based on lean body mass. However, the estimated lean body mass (dry weight) is used if the patient is obese or if there has been a spurious weight gain caused by edema, ascites, or other forms of abnormal fluid retention. It is recommended that before treatment each patient be carefully evaluated to estimate as accurately as possible the optimum initial dosage of fluorouracil. Regardless, the total daily dose is not to exceed 800 mg.

Adult

Usual dose is 12 mg/kg/day given intravenously for 4 consecutive days up to 800 mg daily. If no toxicity is observed, 6 mg/kg are given on days 6,8,10, and 12 unless toxicity occurs. No therapy is given on days 5,7,9, or 11. Therapy is to be discontinued at the end of day 12, even if no toxicity has become apparent. This is followed by weekly maintenance doses, unless toxicity develops.

Poor risk patients or those who are not in an adequate nutritional state should receive 6 mg/kg/day for 3 days. If no toxicity is observed, 3 mg/kg may be given on days 5,7, and 9 unless toxicity occurs. No therapy is given on days 4,6, or 8. The total daily dose should not exceed 400 mg.

A sequence of injections on either schedule constitutes a "course of therapy."

Maintenance therapy:

In instances where toxicity has not been a problem, it is recommended that therapy be continued using either of the following schedules:

1. Repeat dosage of the first course every 30 days after the last day of the previous course of treatment.
2. When toxic signs resulting from the initial course of therapy have subsided, administer a maintenance dosage of 10-15 mg/kg/week as a single dose. Do not exceed 1 gm per week.

High-dose fluorouracil therapy (1-2 gm/day) is routinely given; please consult primary sources in the literature for exact doses and schedules given to specific patient populations. Doses of 20-25 mg/kg have been associated with severe toxicity and death from hemorrhagic colitis or bone marrow failure.

Pediatric

Safety and effectiveness in children have not been well established.

ADMINISTRATION

Intravenous: When given *intravenous push* in the side port of a running line, avoid extravasation; verify venous patency before, during, and after infusion. Rate of injection is not crucial. Flush line completely after infusion. *Continuous infusions* of fluorouracil are added to a convenient volume of D_5W or normal saline and can be administered over 24 hours. Monitor IV site carefully for extravasation; do not administer any other agents through the same line.

Topical: Apply cream BID for 2-4 weeks, or 5% cream BID for 3-6 weeks.

Intraarterial and intracavitary: Refer to original clinical trials for dose and schedules effectively used for specific carcinomas.

Oral: Investigational use only.

STABILITY

Available 50 mg/ml-100 ml vial and 50 mg/ml-50 ml vial. Protect from light. Store at room temperature (15°-

30°C or 59°-86°F). Discoloration (normally colorless to faint yellow) denotes decomposition.

DRUG INTERACTIONS

• Incompatible with diazepam and droperidol.

SIDE EFFECTS AND TOXICITIES

Hematologic

Myelosuppression (dose-limiting) including anemia, leukopenia, thrombocytopenia, and eosinophilia; nadir at 9-14 days for granulocytes and 7-14 days for platelets; recovery by 21 days; toxicity is augmented when combined with leucovorin calcium therapy; epistaxis.

Gastrointestinal

Nausea and vomiting (severity is dose-dependent), anorexia, stomatitis, esophagitis, proctitis, severe diarrhea; GI hemorrhage leading to death.

Renal

Renal failure.

Cardiotoxic

Cardiac arrhythmias, myocardial ischemia, myocardial infarctions, cardiogenic shock, electrocardiographic changes, and angina.

Neurologic

Headache, minor visual disturbances, cerebellar ataxia, lethargy, malaise, and weakness.

Dermatologic

Alopecia (thinning), hyperpigmentation of skin over face, hands, and veins used for infusion, and a pruritic maculopapular rash on the extremities; sun exposure tends to initiate and/or increase skin reactions; "hand-foot syndrome" depicted by painful, erythematous desquamation and fissures of palms and soles.

Hypersensitivities

As with any drug, hypersensitive/allergic/anaphylactic reactions are possible.

Reproductive

The drug has demonstrated mutagenic and teratogenic properties.

Miscellaneous

Photophobia, conjunctivitis, oculomotor dysfunction, blurred vision, and increased lacrimation (the drug is excreted in tears).

WARNINGS/PRECAUTIONS

- Pregnancy category D. It is not known if fluorouracil is excreted in human milk.
- Contraindicated in patients with hepatic and renal disease, bone marrow depression, known hypersensitivity, poor nutritional status, serious infections, angina.
- Severe toxicities and fatalities have occurred in reasonably healthy individuals.

SPECIAL CONSIDERATIONS

- Dosages should be reduced in patients with impaired liver function.
- Preclinical studies have shown that antineoplastic activity of fluorouracil can be potentiated by reduced folates, such as leucovorin calcium. However, severe and fatal adverse effects have been seen with the combination.
- Patients with familial pyrimidinermia should not receive fluorouracil because of the incidence of severe neurotoxicity.

Selected Readings

Ensley JF, Patel B, Kloner R, Ish JA, Wynne J, al-Sarraf M. The clinical syndrome of 5-fluorouracil cardiotoxicity. *Invest New Drugs.* 1989;**7**(1):101-109.

Jakubowski AA, Kemeny N. Hypotension as a manifestation of cardiotoxicity in three patients receiving cisplatin and 5-fluorouracil. *Cancer.* 1988;**62**(2):266-269.

Lomeo AM, Avolio C, Iacobellis G, Manzione L. 5-Fluorouracil cardiotoxicity. *Eur J Gynaecol Oncol.* 1990;**11**(3):237-241.

Mancuso L. Prinzmetal's angina during 5-fluorouracil chemotherapy. *Ann J Med.* 1987;**83**(3):602.

Misset B, Escudier B, Leclercq G, Rivara D, Rougier P, Nitenberg G. Acute myocardiotoxicity during 5-fluorouracil therapy. *Intensive Care Med.* 1990;**16**(3):210-211.

Idarubicin HCl

IDAMYCIN®, IDA, 4-DMDR, 4-demethoxy-daunorubicin

MECHANISM OF ACTION

An anthracycline antibiotic, idarubicin HCl inhibits DNA synthesis by intercalating with DNA, and may inhibit topoisomerase II enzymes. Analog of daunomycin. Cell cycle specific for the S phase.

METABOLISM/EXCRETION

Idarubicin HCl is excreted primarily by hepatobiliary route and to a lesser extent by renal excretion. Half-life: 6-9.4 hours.

INDICATIONS

1. Acute myeloid leukemia (AML)*
2. Chronic myelogenous leukemia (blast phase)
3. Acute lymphocytic leukemia

DOSAGE AND SCHEDULE

Adult

For induction therapy in AML patients the following dose schedule is recommended: IDAMYCIN 12 mg/m²/day for 3 days IV in combination with Ara-C. The Ara-C may be given as 100 mg/m²/day by continuous infusion for 7 days or as Ara-C 25 mg/m² IV bolus followed by Ara-C 200 mg/m²/day by continuous infusion for 5 days. In patients with unequivocal evidence of leukemia after the first induction course, a second course may be administered. Administration of the second course should be delayed in patients who experience severe mucositis, until recovery from this toxicity has occurred, and a dose reduction of 25% is recommended. In patients with hepatic and/or renal impairment, a dose reduction of IDAMYCIN should be considered. IDAMYCIN should not be administered if the bilirubin level exceeds 5%mg.

The benefit of consolidation in prolonging the duration of remissions and survival have not been proven. There is no consensus regarding the optional regimens to be used for consolidation.

Pediatric

Safety and effectiveness in children have not been established.

ADMINISTRATION

Intravenously into the tubing of a free flowing intravenous solution of normal saline or D₅W slowly over 10-15 minutes. Use a large vein. *Vesicant properties.*

STABILITY

Available in 5 mg and 10 mg vials. Reconstituted

solution is stable for 7 days refrigerated and 3 days at room temperature.

DRUG INTERACTIONS
• Incompatible with heparin; precipitation occurs.

SIDE EFFECTS/TOXICITIES

Hematologic
Bone marrow suppression (dose limiting); leukopenia and thrombocytopenia nadir occurs 10-14 days, with recovery in 1-2 weeks.

Gastrointestinal
Mucositis, nausea, vomiting (mild), anorexia, diarrhea and abdominal pain, enterocolitis with bowel perforation; a decrease in hepatic function with elevation in liver enzymes; dose reductions for elevated bilirubin.

Renal
Hyperuricemia and a decrease in renal function.

Cardiac
Congestive heart failure, cardiomyopathy, arrhythmias (atrial fib, chest pain, myocardial infarctions, and other EKG changes), and a decrease in left ventricular ejection fraction. Cardiac toxicity can be fatal; the cardiotoxic effects of idarubicin HCl are similar to that of doxorubicin and daunomycin.

Dermatologic
Alopecia, rash, anthracycline flare reaction, radiation recall reaction, increased sensitivity to sunlight; severe local tissue necrosis if the drug is infiltrated.

Hypersensitivities
As with all drugs, hypersensitive/allergic reactions and anaphylaxis may occur.

Reproductive
Permanent or transient gonadal dysfunction and infertility.

Secondary Neoplasias
The drug may be carcinogenic and/or mutagenic.

WARNINGS/PRECAUTIONS
• Cardiotoxicity is a dose-limiting toxicity of the drug. Unlike the other anthracyclines, the maximum dose of idarubicin that may be administered safely and not cause a decrease in cardiac function is unknown.

- Prior treatment with anthracyclines or cardiotoxic agents, or a preexisting cardiac condition, or prior radiation to the mediastinal area can increase the risk of developing cardiotoxicity to idarubicin HCl. The benefits of treatment with idarubicin HCl should clearly outweigh the risk.
- Monitor renal and hepatic function. Dose reductions are recommended for altered renal and hepatic function.
- Pregnancy category D. It is not known if the drug is excreted in human milk.

SPECIAL CONSIDERATIONS

- Alkalinization of the urine, allopurinol, and intravenous hydration should be started before administration of idarubicin to protect against tumor lysis syndrome.
- Care during administration of drug to avoid extravasation. Extravasation of the drug may occur even in the presence of a blood return and no complaints of pain. Stop the administration of idarubicin immediately if there is any sign or symptom of extravasation. The remainder of the drug may be given in another vein. Ice packs should be applied, the extremity elevated, plastic surgeon consult initiated, and close follow-up of the area is recommended.
- Monitor cardiac function before (baseline) and throughout treatment.
- Patients should be advised to avoid the sun and wear sun protection with an SPF greater than 15.

Selected Readings

Arlin ZA. Idarubicin in acute leukemia: An effective new therapy for the future. *Semin Oncol.* 1989;**16**(1, suppl 2): 35-36.

Berman E, Heller G, Santorsa J, et al. Results of a randomized trial comparing idarubicin and cytosine arabinoside with daunorubicin and cytosine arabinoside in adult patients with newly diagnosed actue myelogenous leukemia. *Blood.* 1991;**77**(8):1666-1674.

Berman E, Raymond V, Gee T, et al. Idarubicin in acute leukemia: Results of studies at Memorial Sloan-Kettering Cancer Center. *Semin Oncol.* 1989b:**16**(1, suppl 2):30-34.

Lambertenghi-Deliliers G, Annaioro C, Cortelezzi A, et al. Idarubicin plus cytarabine as first-line treatment of acute nonlymphoblastic leukemia. *Semin Oncol.* 1989;**16**(2, suppl 2):16-20.

Wiernik PH, Case DC Jr, Periman PO, et al. A multicenter trial of cytarabine plus idarubicin or daunorubicin as induction therapy for adult nonlymphocytic leukemia. *Semin Oncol.* 1989;**16**(1, suppl 2):25-29.

Ifosfamide

IFEX®, isophosphamide

MECHANISM OF ACTION

Alkylating agent with cell cycle nonspecific properties. A structural analog of cyclophosphamide. Activated by microsomes in the liver. Ifosfamide destroys DNA by binding to protein, DNA cross-linking, and inhibition of DNA synthesis.

METABOLISM/EXCRETION

The drug is extensively and variably metabolized in the liver. Much of the drug (70%-80%) is excreted in the urine unchanged. Half-life ranges from 3-10 hours for low-dose therapy to 13.8 hours for high-dose therapy.

INDICATIONS

1. When used in combination with certain chemotherapeutic agents, it is indicated for third-line germ cell testicular cancer*
2. Bone and soft tissue sarcomas
3. Ewing's sarcoma
4. Non-Hodgkin's lymphoma
5. Lung cancer
6. Pancreatic sarcoma

DOSAGE AND SCHEDULE

Adult

IFEX should be administered intravenously at a dose of 1.2 gm/m²/day for 5 consecutive days. Treatment is repeated every 3 weeks or after recovery from hematologic toxicity (platelets ≥ 100,00/mm³, WBC ≥ 4,000/mm³). To prevent bladder toxicity, IFEX should be given with extensive hydration consisting of at least 2 liters of oral or intravenous fluid per day. A protector, such as mesna, should also be used to prevent hemorrhagic cystitis. IFEX should be administered as a

slow infusion lasting a minimum of 30 minutes.
Although IFEX has been administered to a small
number of patients with compromised hepatic and/or
renal function, studies to establish optimal dose
schedules of IFEX in such patients have not been
conducted.

Pediatric

Safety and effectiveness in children have not been well
established.

ADMINISTRATION

Intravenous: Usually as a short infusion, over 30
minutes. May be given slow IV push in a minimum of
75 ml of sterile saline, NOT WATER. *Continuous
infusion* over 5 days. Compatible solutions include
0.9% sodium chloride, 5% dextrose in water, and
lactated ringer's solution. Ifosphamide is compatible
with mesna for up to 9 days at temperatures up to
27°C.

STABILITY

Available in 1 gm and 3 gm vials. Stable if stored at
room temperature or under refrigeration for long periods
of time. Temperatures above 35°C may cause
liquification of the drug and accelerate decomposition.
When diluted with bacteriostatic water with benzyl
alcohol or parabens and under refrigeration, the vial is
stable for 1 week. Otherwise, diluted drug is stable for 8
hours.

DRUG INTERACTIONS

• Allopurinol, cimetidine, phenobarbital, phenytoin,
  chloral hydrate, chloroquine, phenothiazides,
  potassium iodide, chloramphenicol, imipramine,
  vitamin A, corticosteroids, and succinylcholine may
  effect the activity and/or the toxicity of ifosfamide.

SIDE EFFECTS AND TOXICITIES

Hematologic

Dose-limiting myelosuppression; granulocytes nadir in
10-14 days, recovery in 21 days; thrombocytopenia and
anemia.

Gastrointestinal

Nausea and vomiting; severity is dose- and schedule-
dependent with an onset in 3-6 hours, and a duration

up to 3 days. Mucositis, hepatic toxicity, diarrhea, or constipation; anorexia.

Renal
Urotoxicity is the dose-limiting adverse effect; hemorrhagic cystitis, dysuria, urinary frequency, and bladder irritation could be prevented with uroprotection (mesna, ascorbic acid, or Mucomyst) and hydration; symptoms of renal toxicity, including increased BUN and serum creatinine, decreased urine CrCl, acute tubular necrosis, pyelonephritis, glomerular dysfunction, and metabolic acidosis all may result if the bladder is not adequately flushed and protected.

Neurologic
Lethargy, ataxia, stupor, weakness, facial paresthesia, somnolence, confusion, dizziness, depressive psychosis, hallucinations, disorientation, seizures, cranial nerve dysfunction, and coma. Incidence may be higher in patients receiving high doses of ifosfamide and those with impaired renal function.

Dermatologic
Alopecia, hyperpigmentation and nail ridging, dermatitis, phlebitis, and skin necrosis.

Hypersensitivity
As with all drugs, hypersensitive/allergic reactions and anaphylaxis may occur.

Reproductive
Infertility is common.

Secondary Neoplasias
The drug has demonstrated mutagenic, teratogenic, and carcinogenic properties.

WARNINGS/PRECAUTIONS
- Contraindicated in patients with severely depressed bone marrow, previous hypersensitivity to ifosfamide, and patients with renal disease.
- Pregnancy category D. The drug is excreted in human milk.

SPECIAL CONSIDERATIONS
- Adequate hydration before and 72 hours after therapy (minimum 2 l/day) is necessary to reduce the incidence of drug-induced hemorrhagic cystitis.

- Administer ifosfamide with a uroprotector (e.g., mesna).
- The use of mesna is required for high-dose ifosfamide therapy.

Selected Readings

Klein HO, Dias Wickramanayake P, Coerper CL, et al. High dose ifosfamide and mesna as continuous infusion over five days—A phrase I/II trial. *Cancer Treat Rev.* 1983;**10**(suppl A):167-173.

Loehrer PJ, Einhorn LH, Williams SD. VP-16 plus ifosfamide plus cisplatin as salvage therapy in refractory germ cell cancer. *J Clin Oncol.* 1986;**4**:528-536.

Shaw IC, Rose JW. Infusion of ifosfamide plus mesna. *Lancet.* 1984;**1**:1353-1354.

Zalupski M, Baker LH. Ifosfamide. *J Natl Cancer Inst.* 1988;**80**:556-566.

Lomustine

CCNU, CeeNU®

MECHANISM OF ACTION

An alkylating agent (nitrosourea) that is cell cycle nonspecific. Lomustine inhibits RNA and DNA synthesis through alkylation and may inhibit key enzymatic processes by carbamoylation of amino acids in proteins.

METABOLISM/EXCRETION

Rapid oral absorption. The high lipid solubility of lomustine facilitates transport across the blood brain barrier. The serum half-life of the metabolites ranges from 16 hours to 2 days. Urinary excretion is slow. About 60% of a dose is recovered after 48 hours, with 50% recovered within the first 12-24 hours.

INDICATIONS

1. Brain tumors* (primary or metastatic)
2. Hodgkin's disease*
3. Multiple myeloma
4. Gastrointestinal carcinoma
5. Non-small cell lung carcinoma (advanced)

DOSAGE AND SCHEDULE

Adult and Pediatric

The recommended dose of CeeNU in adults and children as a single agent in previously untreated patients is 130 mg/m^2 as a single oral dose every 6 weeks. In individuals with compromised bone marrow function, the dose should be reduced to 100 mg/m^2 every 6 weeks. When CeeNU is used in combination with other myelosuppressive drugs, the doses should be adjusted accordingly. Doses subsequent to the initial dose should be adjusted according to the hematologic response of the patient to the preceding dose. See manufacturer guide to dosage adjustment.

A repeat course of CeeNU should not be given until circulating blood elements have returned to acceptable levels (platelets above 100,000/mm^3; leukocytes above 4000/mm^3) and this is usually in 6 weeks. Adequate number of neutrophils should be present on a peripheral blood smear. Blood counts should be monitored weekly and repeat courses should not be given before 6 weeks because the hematologic toxicity is delayed and cumulative.

ADMINISTRATION
Oral: Take on an empty stomach at bedtime.

STABILITY
Capsules come in the following strengths: 100 mg (green/green), 40 mg (white/green), 10 mg (white/white). Lomustine is stored at room temperature in closed containers. Avoid exposure to moisture and protect from excessive heat (> 40°C). Expiration dates are indicated on the package labeling.

DRUG INTERACTIONS
- Cimetidine has been shown to potentiate lomustine myelotoxicity.
- Consumption of alcohol should be avoided for a short period following lomustine.

SIDE EFFECTS AND TOXICITIES
Hematologic
Delayed and cumulative myelosuppression is the dose-limiting toxicity; thrombocytopenia nadir in 4 weeks, lasts 1-2 weeks; leukopenia nadir 5-6 weeks, lasts 1-2 weeks; thrombocytopenia may be more severe than leukopenia; anemia.

Gastrointestinal
Nausea and vomiting can occur 2-6 hours and last about

24 hours. Anorexia, diarrhea and stomatitis. Hepatic toxicity is manifested by increased transaminase, alkaline phosphatase, bilirubin, and jaundice.

Renal

Nephrotoxicity, evidenced by progressive azotemia, decrease in kidney size, and renal failure; renal failure may be fatal; damage to the kidneys may occur at lower doses.

Pulmonary

Pulmonary fibrosis and/or pulmonary infiltrates may occur months after the start of treatment; pulmonary toxicity is more common in patients receiving cumulative doses greater than 1100 mg/m^2, but can occur at much lower doses. Treatment with related nitrosoureas in combination with cranial radiation has led to the development of pulmonary fibrosis, which may occur years later.

Neurologic

Confusion, ataxia, lethargy and dysarthria. Patients treated with low dose cranial irradiation and lomustine have developed permanent cortical blindness.

Dermatologic

Alopecia.

Hypersensitivities

Contraindicated in patients with a previous hypersensitivity; as with all drugs, hypersensitive/allergic reactions and anaphylaxis may occur.

Reproductive

May impair fertility.

Secondary Neoplasias

Long-term use of nitrosoureas have been associated with the development of secondary malignancies; the drug has teratogenic, mutagenic, and carcinogenic properties.

Miscellaneous

Ocular damage: optic neuritis, retinopathy, and blurred vision.

WARNINGS/PRECAUTIONS

- Hematologic monitoring is required for at least 6 weeks after a dose. Dose adjustments may be required for nadir blood counts. Doses should not be repeated earlier than every 6 weeks.
- Pulmonary function tests should be obtained at

baseline and during treatment. Patients with a baseline below 70% of the predicted Forced Vital Capacity or Carbon Monoxide Diffusing Capacity are at risk of developing pulmonary toxicity.
- Pregnancy category D. It is not known if lomustine is excreted in human milk.

SPECIAL CONSIDERATIONS
- Patients should be informed that capsules come in various strengths and colors and that treatment is a single dose repeated no sooner than every 6 weeks.

Selected Readings

Brusamolino E, Pagnucco G, Castelli G, et al. The risk of secondary myelodysplasia and acute non-lymphoid leukemia in Hodgkin's disease is related to combined modality therapy and to the use of nitrosourea derivatives. *Proc Am Soc Clin Oncol.* 1992;**11**:329.

Hansen HH, Selawry OS, Pajak TF, et al. The superiority of CCNU in the treatment of advanced Hodgkin's disease: Cancer and leukemia group B study. *Cancer.* 1981;**47**:14-18.

Lefkowitz IB, Packer RJ, SuttonLN, et al. Results of the treatment of children with recurrent gliomas with lomustine and vincristine. *Cancer.* 1988;**61**:896-902.

Vats TS, Trueworthy RC, Langston CM. Pulmonary fibrosis associated with lomustine (CCNU): A case report. *Cancer Treat Rep.* 1982;**66**(10):1881-1882.

Mechlorethamine HCl

Mustargen®, nitrogen mustard, NH2

MECHANISM OF ACTION

Cell cycle nonspecific alkylating agent. Analog of mustard gas which forms a highly reactive carbonium ion that causes intrastrand and interstrand cross-linkage and base pairing of DNA. Interferes with DNA replication, RNA, and protein synthesis.

METABOLISM/EXCRETION

There is a rapid transformation to metabolites; within minutes the drug cannot be detected in the blood. Modest amounts (0.01%) are excreted unchanged in the urine; 50% of the inactive metabolites are excreted within 24 hours.

INDICATIONS
1. Stages III and IV Hodgkin's disease* and non-Hodgkin's lymphoma*
2. Lymphosarcoma
3. Chronic myelocytic* or lymphocytic* leukemia
4. Polycythemia vera
5. Mycosis fungoides*
6. Bronchogenic carcinoma*
7. Intrapleural, intrapericardial, and intraperitoneal palliative treatment of metastatic carcinoma resulting in effusion

DOSAGE AND SCHEDULE
Adult
Intravenous:

The dosage of Mustargen varies with the clinical situation, the therapeutic response, and the magnitude of hematologic depression.

A total dose of 0.4 mg/kg of body weight for each course usually is given either as a single dose or in divided doses of 0.1-0.2 mg/kg/day. Dosage should be based on ideal dry body weight. The presence of edema or ascites must be considered so that the dosage will be based on actual weight unaugmented by these conditions.

The margin of safety in therapy with Mustargen is narrow and considerable care must be exercised in the manner of dosage. Repeated examinations of blood counts are *mandatory* as a guide to subsequent therapy.

Subsequent courses should not be given until the patient has recovered hematologically from the previous course; this is best determined by repeated studies of the peripheral blood elements awaiting their return to normal levels. It is often possible to give repeated courses of Mustargen as early as 3 weeks after treatment.

MOPP regimen uses 6 mg/m^2 on days 1 and 8 of a 14-day chemotherapeutic regimen.

Intracavitary:

Nitrogen mustard has been used by intracavitary administration with varying success in certain malignant conditions for the control of pleural, peritoneal, and pericardial effusions made by malignant cells.

The usual dose of nitrogen mustard for intracavitary injection is 0.4 mg/kg of body weight, though 0.2 mg/kg (or, 10-20 mg) has been used by the intrapericardial route. The position of the patient should be changed every 5-10 minutes for an hour after injection to obtain more uniform distribution of the drug throughout the serous cavity. Remaining fluid may be removed from the pleural or peritoneal cavity by paracentesis 24-36 hours later. Patients should be followed carefully by clinical and x-ray examination to detect reaccumulation of fluid.

Pediatric

Use in children has been limited. Safety and effectiveness have not been published in well-controlled studies. It has been administered to children as part of the MOPP regimen.

ADMINISTRATION

Mechlorethamine HCl is a vesicant and should be prepared and administered with the utmost caution.
Mechlorethamine HCl is administered IV push through the sideport of a running D_5W or normal saline infusion line. Venous patency should be confirmed before, during, and after administration.

STABILITY

Available in 10 mg vials. It is advised to use the drug within 15-30 minutes of mixing; since the manufacturer reports 15 minutes of stability after reconstitution.

DRUG INTERACTIONS

• May reduce effectiveness of antigout medications through raising uric acid levels.

SIDE EFFECTS AND TOXICITIES

Hematologic

Myelosuppression is dose-limiting; granulocyte nadir in 1 week, with recovery in 10 days to 3 weeks; thrombocytopenia is variable with a time course similar to granulocytopenia; platelet depression may be severe and patients may experience bleeding from the gums and GI tract, petechiae, and small subcutaneous hemorrhages; persistent pancytopenia and severe uncontrollable depression of the hematopoietic system.

Gastrointestinal

Nausea and vomiting are universal and severe, beginning within the first 3 hours and lasting 4-8 hours, but may persist up to 24 hours; anorexia, diarrhea and colitis, weight loss, stomatitis and jaundice; metallic taste immediately after therapy.

Renal

Hyperuricemia

Neurologic

Weakness, sleepiness, dizziness, paresthesia, peripheral neuropathies, tinnitus, diminished hearing, temporary aphasia and paresis, and headache; CNS toxicities are more common and severe if mechlorethamine HCl is administered via the intracarotid artery.

Dermatologic

Mechlorethamine is a vesicant, and severe painful inflammation, erythema, induration, and necrosis are likely if extravasation occurs; alopecia, puritus, maculopapular skin eruptions, and herpes zoster.

Hypersensitivities

Severe allergic reactions including anaphylaxis are rare, but may occur.

Reproductive

Amenorrhea (temporary or permanent), delayed menses, oligomenorrhea, azoospermia, impaired spermatogenesis, and total germinal aplasia.

Secondary Neoplasias

Secondary neoplasias and various chromosomal abnormalities are possible.

WARNINGS/PRECAUTIONS

- Extravasation into subcutaneous tissue will cause a painful inflammation. The area can become indurated and sloughing may occur.
- Pregnancy category D. It is not known if the drug is excreted in human milk.
- The use of mechlorethamine HCl is contraindicated in patients with prior anaphylactic reactions to mechlorethamine and in those with active infectious diseases.

SPECIAL CONSIDERATIONS

- Extravasation into subcutaneous tissue will cause a

painful inflammation. The area can become indurated and sloughing may occur. Treating the extravasated area with sodium thiosulfate and cold compresses is a recommended antidote (see manufacturer and institutional policy and procedure guidelines for specific antidotal therapy).

Selected Readings

Anderson CB, Philpott GW, Ferguson TB. The treatment of malignant pleural effusions. *Cancer.* 1974;**33:**916-922.

Fracchia A, Knaper W, Carey J, Farrow J. Intrapleural chemotherapy for effusion from metastatic breast carcinoma. *Cancer.* 1970;**26:**626-629.

Leininger B, Barker W, Langston H. A simplified method for management of malignant pleural effusion. *J Thorac Cardiovasc Surg.* 1969;**58**(5):758-763.

Melphalan

Alkeran®, Phenylalanine mustard, L-sarcolysin, L-PAM

MECHANISM OF ACTION

Cell cycle nonspecific alkylating agent. Derivative of nitrogen mustard. Primary effect on DNA. The alkylation process is bifunctional and involves cross-linking of DNA strands in both resting and rapidly dividing tumor cells.

METABOLISM/EXCRETION

Metabolized by spontaneous hydrolysis in plasma. Melphalan is poorly absorbed if taken with food. Oral absorption is both erratic and incomplete, peaking in 2 hours. Absolute oral bioavailability ranges between 25% to 89% with a mean of 56%. The intravenous drug appears to have a biphasic elimination with a half-life of 6-8 minutes and 40-60 minutes. The majority of the drug appears to be cleared by nonrenal mechanisms, with 25%-50% excreted in the feces over 6 days and 25%-30% in the urine within 24 hours.

INDICATIONS

1. Multiple myeloma* (for whom oral therapy is not appropriate); approved intravenous indication is for

patients with multiple myeloma who require
palliative treatment for whom oral therapy is not
appropriate
2. Breast and ovarian* carcinomas
3. Testicular carcinoma
4. Intravenous formulation has shown activity in
   sarcomas, rhabdomyosarcoma, Ewing's sarcoma,
   and non-small cell lung cancer

DOSAGE AND SCHEDULE
Adult
Multiple myeloma:

The usual oral dose is 6 mg/day (3 tablets). The entire
daily dose may be given at one time. It is adjusted, as
required, on the basis of blood counts done at
approximately weekly intervals. After 2-3 weeks of
treatment, the drug should be discontinued for up to 4
weeks during which time the blood count should be
followed carefully. When the WBC and platelet counts
are rising, a maintenance dose of 2 mg/day may be
instituted. Because of the patient-to-patient variation in
melphalan plasma levels following oral administration
of the drug, it has been recommended that melphalan
dosage be cautiously escalated until some
myelosuppression is observed, to assure that potentially
therapeutic levels of the drug have been reached.

Other dosage regimens have been used. One initial
course gives 10 mg/day for 7-10 days. With this
regimen maximal suppression of the leukocyte and
platelet count occurs within 3-5 weeks and recovery
within 4-8 weeks. Continuous maintenance therapy
with 2 mg/day is instituted when the WBC is greater
than 4,000/mm^3 and the platelet count is greater than
100,000/mm^3. Dosage is adjusted to between 1-3
mg/day depending upon the hematologic response. It is
desirable to try to maintain a significant degree of bone
marrow depression so as to keep the leukocyte count in
the range of 3,000-3,500 cells/mm^3. Another regimen
starts with 0.15 mg/kg/day for 7 days. This is followed
by a rest period of at least 14 days, but it may be as
long as 5-6 weeks. Maintenance therapy is started when
the WBC and platelet counts are rising. The

maintenance dose is 0.05 mg/kg/day or less and is adjusted according to the blood count.

It has been reported that the use of melphalan in combination with prednisone significantly improves the percentage of patients with multiple myeloma who achieve palliation. One regimen has been to administer courses of melphalan at 0.25 mg/kg/day for 4 days (or, 0.20 mg/kg/day for 5 days), for a total dose of 1 mg/kg per course. These 4- or 5-day courses are repeated every 4-6 weeks if the granulocyte count and the platelet count have returned to normal levels. It is to be emphasized that response may be very gradual over many months; it is important that repeated courses or continuous therapy be given, since improvement may continue slowly over several months and the maximum benefit may be missed if the treatment is stopped too soon.

In patients with moderate to severe renal impairment, currently available pharmacokinetic data do not justify an absolute recommendation on dosage reduction to those patients, but it may be prudent to use a reduced dose initially.

Epithelial ovarian carcinoma:
One commonly employed regimen for the treatment of ovarian carcinoma has been to administer melphalan at a dose of 0.2 mg/kg/day for 5 days as a single course. Courses are repeated every 4-5 weeks depending upon hematologic tolerance.

Single course of PO 0.2 mg/kg/day in divided doses for 5 days. The course may be repeated every 4-5 weeks depending on hematologic tolerance.

Pediatric
The safety and effectiveness in children have not been established.

ADMINISTRATION
Oral: 2 mg tablets. *Intravenous* formulation (investigational use) should be given as a slow infusion in 100-200 ml D_5W or normal saline over 15-45 minutes. IV drug is an *irritant.* May be given by continuous infusion; check stability carefully.

STABILITY
Store tablets (2 mg/tab) at room temperature.

DRUG INTERACTIONS

- Cyclosporin increases the risk of nephrotoxicity.
- Misonidazole enhances DNA cross-linking from melphalan and thereby increases the agent's cytotoxicity as well.
- Corticosteroids may enhance the antitumor effects of melphalan.
- Cimetidine decreases melphalan's oral bioavailability by approximately 30%.

SIDE EFFECTS AND TOXICITIES

Hematologic

Bone marrow depression (anemia, leukopenia, agranulocytosis, and thrombocytopenia) nadirs in 14-21 days; there may be a delayed onset, with a cumulative nadir 4-6 weeks after therapy; chronic thrombocytopenia.

Gastrointestinal

Nausea and vomiting are mild with low-dose and continuous-dose schedules, and severe with high-dose therapy; anorexia, stomatitis, hepatic toxicity including veno-occlusive disease.

Pulmonary

Bronchopulmonary dysplasia and pulmonary fibrosis.

Dermatologic

Alopecia, infrequent urticaria and/or a maculopapular rash; skin ulcerations at the injection site, skin necrosis, and vasculitis with the intravenous formulation.

Hypersensitivity

IV melphalan can cause anaphylaxis, diaphoresis, hypotension, tachycardia, bronchospasm, dyspnea, and cardiac arrest; anaphylaxis with oral melphalan (rare).

Reproductive

Melphalan may cause fetal harm when administered to pregnant women.

Secondary Neoplasias

Acute nonlymphatic leukemia; acute myelogenous leukemia and myelodysplasia with long-term oral dosing; drug is potentially mutagenic and teratogenic.

WARNINGS/PRECAUTIONS

- Consider dose reductions on patients with renal insufficiency receiving IV melphalan.

- Contraindicated in patients who have experienced hypersensitivity to this agent.
- Pregnancy category D. It is not known if melphalan is excreted in human milk.
- Caution should be used with the concurrent use of chemotherapy and radiation therapy, and in patients with severe anemia, neutropenia, thrombocytopenia, and impaired renal function.

SPECIAL CONSIDERATIONS

- IV melphalan can cause serious hypersensitivity reactions.
- Total daily dose should be taken at once on an empty stomach.
- Use an aggressive antiemetic regimen with intravenous melphalan.
- Treat IV melphalan as an irritant during its administration.

Selected Readings

Codling BW, Chakera TMH. Pulmonary fibrosis following therapy with melphalan for multiple myeloma. *J Clin Pathol.* 1972;**25**:668-673.

Einhorn N. Acute leukemia after chemotherapy (melphalan). *Cancer.* 1978;**44**:444-447.

Lawrence BV, Harvey HA, Lipton A. Anaphylaxis due to oral melphalan (letter). *Cancer Treat Rep.* 1980;**64**(4/5):731-732.

Selby PJ, Millal Jl, Phelps TA, et al. The combination of melphalan with prednisolone. Anti-tumor effect and normal tissue toxicity in laboratory systems. *Cancer Chemother Pharmacol.* 1981;**6**:169-173.

6-Mercaptopurine

Purinethol®, mercaptopurine, 6-MP

MECHANISM OF ACTION

Antimetabolite ("false") purine antagonist. When converted into monophosphate nucleotides, it inhibits de novo protein synthesis, and by competing with endogenous ribotides it can halt RNA synthesis. Cell cycle S specific.

METABOLISM/EXCRETION

Metabolized in the liver and kidney by the enzyme
xanthine oxidase. Fifty percent of the drug is excreted in
the urine (11% in the first 6 hours). Half-life IV: 20-50
minutes, PO: 1-2 hours. Oral bioavailability is low.

INDICATIONS

1. Acute lymphatic leukemia in children and adults
   (POMP)*
2. Second line therapy in chronic granulocytic
   leukemia*
3. Chronic myelogenous leukemia*(maintenance and
   primary therapy)
4. Refractory solid tumors
5. Histiocytic and undifferentiated lymphomas
6. Pediatric non-Hodgkin's lymphoma (combination
   therapy)
7. As an immunosuppressant for Crohn's disease

DOSAGE AND SCHEDULE

Adult and Pediatric

Induction therapy:

Purinethol (mercaptopurine) is administered orally.
The dosage that will be tolerated and effective varies
from patient to patient; therefore, careful titration is
necessary to obtain the optimum therapeutic effect
without incurring excessive, unintended toxicity. The
usual initial dosage for children and adults is 2.5
mg/kg/day (100-200 mg in the average adult and 50
mg in an average 5-year-old child). Children with
acute leukemia have tolerated this dose without
difficulty in most cases; it may be continued daily for
several weeks or more in some patients. If after 4
weeks at this dosage there is no clinical improvement
and no definite evidence of leukocyte or platelet
depression, the dosage may be increased up to 5
mg/kg/day. A dosage of 2.5 mg/kg/day may result in a
rapid fall in leukocyte count within 1 to 2 weeks in
some adults with acute lymphatic leukemia and high
total leukocyte counts. The total daily dose may be
given at one time. It is calculated to the nearest
multiple of 25 mg. *The dosage of mercaptopurine
should be reduced to one third to one quarter of the*

usual dose if allopurinol is given concurrently.
Because the drug may have a delayed action, it should
be discontinued at the first sign of an abnormally large
or rapid fall in the leukocyte count or platelet count. If
subsequently the leukocyte count or platelet count
remains constant for 2 or 3 days, or rises, treatment
may be resumed.

Maintenance therapy:

Once a complete hematologic remission is obtained,
maintenance therapy is considered essential.
Maintenance doses will vary from patient to patient. A
usual daily maintenance dose of mercaptopurine is 1.5 to
2.5 mg/kg/day as a single dose. In children with acute
lymphatic leukemia in remission, superior results have
been obtained when mercaptopurine has been combined
with other agents (most frequently with methotrexate)
for remission maintenance. Mercaptopurine should
rarely be relied upon as a single agent for the
maintenance of remissions induced in acute leukemia.

ADMINISTRATION

Oral tablet—50 mg, usually administered as a single
daily dose. Investigational (500 mg vials), is given slow
IV push over several minutes. It may also be given as a
continuous infusion over 12-48 hours.

STABILITY

Store tablets at room temperature and protect from light.
   Diluted 6-Mercaptopurine is stable for 4 hours in the
refrigerator.

DRUG INTERACTIONS

• Incompatible with sodium allopurinol and
  prednisolone sodium succinate.
• Concomitant use with allopurinol requires up to a 75%
  dose reduction of 6-Mercaptopurine.
• Antagonizing effect on the anticoagulant properties of
  warfarin. There is complete cross-resistance between
  mercaptopurine and Tabloid brand thioguanine.

SIDE EFFECTS AND TOXICITIES

Hematologic

Myelosuppression is mild; leukopenia (nadir 11-23
days) and thrombocytopenia (nadir 12-21 days); anemia
with high-dose therapy.

Gastrointestinal

Nausea and vomiting are mild and infrequent; anorexia; mucositis and stomatitis with high-dose and continuous infusion therapy; diarrhea, hepatitis, jaundice (may occur 2-3 months after therapy), biliary stasis, cumulative hyperbilirubinemia, elevated alkaline phosphatase and SGOT levels; hepatic necrosis has resulted in death.

Renal

Renal failure, oliguria, hematuria, flank pain, crystalluria (high-dose intravenous therapy), and hyperuricemia with rapid leukemia cell lysis.

Neurologic

Headache.

Dermatologic

Dry-scaling rash, urticaria, and skin eruption.

Hypersensitivities

As with all drugs, hypersensitive/allergic reactions and anaphylaxis may occur.

Reproductive

Mercaptopurine can cause fetal harm when administered to pregnant women, and increase the incidence of first trimester abortions. The effect on fertility is unknown in males and females.

Secondary Neoplasias

Carcinogenic potential exists in man; chromosomal aberrations have been noted.

Miscellaneous

Fever and weakness; mercaptopurine may manifest decreased cellular hypersensitivities and impaired allograft rejection. Induction of immunity to infectious agents or vaccines will be subnormal in these patients. The degree of immunosuppression will depend on antigen dose and temporal relationship to drug.

WARNINGS/PRECAUTIONS

- Contraindicated in patients with known hypersensitivity and prior resistance to 6-Mercaptopurine.
- Pregnancy (category D). It is not known whether the drug is excreted in human milk.
- Use with caution in patients with impaired renal/hepatic function, and concomitantly with

allopurinol. Increased toxicity when given with
radiation and cytotoxic therapy.

SPECIAL CONSIDERATIONS

- Elevations in serum glucose and uric acid may be
  related to 6-Mercaptopurine.
- Use reduced doses in hepatic/renal impairment.

Selected Readings

Duttura MJ, Carolla RL, Gallelli JF, et al. Hematuria and crystalluria
    after high-dose 6-mercaptopurine administration. *N Engl J Med.*
    1972;**287**(6):292-294.
Einhorn M, Davidson I. Hepatoxicity of mercaptopurine. *JAMA.*
    1964;**188**:802-806.
Ellison RR, Hoogstraten B, Holland JF, et al. Intermittent therapy with
    6-mercaptopurine (NSC-755) and methotrexate (NSC-740) given
    intravenously to adults with acute leukemia. *Cancer Chemother
    Rep.* 1972;**56**:535-542.

Methotrexate

MTX, amethopterin, methotrexate sodium, Folex®,
Mexate®, Methotrexate Tablets®, for Injection®, LPF®,
Rheumatrex®

MECHANISM OF ACTION

Cell cycle S phase specific antimetabolite. Action
includes blockade of the enzyme dihydrofolate
reductase (DHFR), which inhibits the conversion of
folic acid to tetrahydrofolic acid which results in the
arrest of DNA, RNA, and protein synthesis.

METABOLISM/EXCRETION

Absorbed in the GI tract, metabolized in the liver. Oral
peaks in 1-4 hours, IV peaks in $1/_2$ - 2 hours. Half-life: 2
hours. Approximately 50%-60% of the drug is found in
the blood; bound to plasma proteins. Almost all of the
drug is excreted unchanged in the urine. Crosses blood
brain and placental barrier.

INDICATIONS

1. Carcinoma of the breast*, head and neck*,
   gastrointestinal, and lung (non-small cell, limited
   small cell*)
2. Osteosarcomas

3. Acute lymphocytic leukemia*
4. Meningeal leukemia* or carcinomatosis
5. Gestational trophoblastic carcinomas; choriocarcinoma*, chorioadenoma destruens*, and hydatidiform mole*
6. Advanced stage non-Hodgkin's lymphoma*
7. Burkitt's lymphoma
8. Mycosis fungoides

DOSAGE AND SCHEDULE

Adult

Choriocarcinoma and similar trophoblastic diseases:

Methotrexate is administered orally or intramuscularly in doses of 15-30 mg/day for a 5-day course. Repeated for 3-5 cycles as required, with rest periods of 1 or more weeks interposed between courses, until any manifesting toxic symptoms subside.

Leukemia:

Methotrexate alone or in combination with steroids was used initially for induction of remission in acute lymphoblastic leukemias. More recently corticosteroid therapy, in combination with other antileukemic drugs or in cyclic combinations with methotrexate, has appeared to produce rapid and effective remissions.

Induction therapy: methotrexate in doses of 3.3 mg/m^2 in combination with prednisone 60 mg/m^2, given daily.

Maintenance therapy: methotrexate is administered two times weekly either by mouth or intramuscularly in total weekly doses of 30 mg/m^2. It has also been given in doses of 2.5 mg/kg intravenously every 14 days.

A variety of combination chemotherapy regimens has been used for both induction and maintenance therapy in acute lymphoblastic leukemia. The physician should be familiar with the new advances in antileukemic therapy.

Lymphomas:

In Burkitt's tumor, Stage I-II, methotrexate has produced prolonged remissions in some cases. Recommended dosage is 10-25 mg/day orally for 4-8 days. In Stage III, methotrexate is commonly given concomitantly with other antitumor agents. Treatment of all stages usually consists of several courses of the

drug interposed with 7-10 day rest periods.
Lymphosarcomas in Stage III may respond to combined
drug therapy with methotrexate given in doses of 0.625
to 2.5 mg/kg/day.

Mycosis fungoides:

Dosage is usually 2.5 to 10 mg/day by mouth for weeks
or months. Dose levels and adjustment of dose regimen
by reduction or cessation of the drug are guided by
patient response and hematologic monitoring.
Methotrexate has also been given intramuscularly in
doses of 50 mg once weekly or 25 mg 2 times weekly.

Osteosarcoma:

An effective adjuvant chemotherapy regimen requires
the administration of several cytotoxic
chemotherapeutic agents. In addition to high-dose
methotrexate with leucovorin rescue, these agents may
include doxorubicin, cisplatin, and the combination of
bleomycin, cyclophosphamide, and dactinomycin-D
(BCD). The starting dose of high-dose methotrexate
treatment is 12 gm/m^2. If this dose is not sufficient to
produce a peak serum methotrexate concentration of
1,000 micromolar at the end of the methotrexate
infusion, the dose may be escalated to 15 gm/m^2 in
subsequent treatments.

*The manufacturer recommends specific safety
guidelines for high-dose methotrexate with leucovorin
rescue. Please refer to the specific guidelines detailed in
the package insert and to the policy and procedures of
your institution.*

Pediatric

Pediatric safety and effectiveness have only been
established in cancer-chemotherapy indications. Dosing
in children has been based on age. We urge referral to
primary literature sources and specific manufacturer
guidelines for specific dose and schedule guidelines.

ADMINISTRATION

Methotrexate may be given by *oral, intravenous
(infusion or push), intrathecal, intramuscular, or
intraarterial routes.* The preserved formulation must not
be given intrathecally or in high-dose therapy. Oral
administration is often preferred when low doses are

being administered, since absorption is rapid and
effective serum levels are obtained.

STABILITY

Available in 2.5 mg tablets and 50 mg (investigational)
for high-dose therapy. Available solution vials (2 ml)
contain 2.5 or 25 mg/ml. Additionally, a 20 mg/20 ml
vial is available for intravenous and intrathecal use, as
well as 100, 500, and 1000 mg vials which do not
contain preservatives. Tablets and intact vials are stable
for 2 years when stored at room temperature.
Reconstituted solutions are stable for 7 days, but should
be discarded after 24 hours.

DRUG INTERACTIONS

- **Do not** use concurrently with cotrimoxazole,
  pyrimethamine, NSAIDS (with high-dose therapy).
- The list of drugs that interact with methotrexate is
  extensive; please refer to the literature for detailed
  explanation of the interactive effects: allopurinol,
  cephalothin, chloramphenicol, dexamethasone,
  hydrocortisone, ketoprofen, penicillin G, phenytoin,
  prednisone, prednisolone, pristinamycin, probenecid,
  salicylate, sulfasoxazole, tetracycline, thymidine,
  tolbutamide, and vincristine.
- Alcohol increases risk of hepatotoxicity.
- Severe reactions occur when live vaccines are given
  with methotrexate.

SIDE EFFECTS AND TOXICITIES

Hematologic

Myelosuppression, nadirs: hemoglobin 6-13 days,
reticulocyte 2-7 days, leukocytes 4-7 days (second phase
12-21 days), and platelets 5-21 days, recovery is rapid.

Gastrointestinal

Nausea and vomiting are dose dependent and may occur
during administration and last 24-72 hours; anorexia,
stomatitis (severe) occur in 3-5 days in high-dose
therapy and 3-4 weeks in low-dose therapy; diarrhea,
cramps, ulcers, melena, hematemesis, enteritis, and
intestinal perforation; hepatotoxicity can lead to
cirrhosis in severe cases.

Renal

Acute renal tubular necrosis, renal failure, urinary

retention, azotemia, and uric acid nephropathy; risks of renal failure may be decreased by alkalinization of the urine.

Pulmonary

Pneumothorax may occur in the first 48 hours after high-dose therapy in patients with pulmonary metastasis; allergic pneumonitis accompanied with eosinophilia, pulmonary infiltrates, fever, cough, and shortness of breath, with high-dose therapy may be fatal; pneumonitis may occur with low-dose therapy.

Neurologic

Dizziness, malaise, blurred vision, and symptoms of increased CSF pressure (seizures, paresis, headache, fever, nausea and vomiting, and brain atrophy), convulsions, Guillain-Barré-like syndrome following intrathecal therapy.

Dermatologic

Alopecia, dermatitis, pruritus, urticaria, dry skin, petechiae, ecchymosis, acne, photosensitivity, and a sunburn-like rash, radiation recall.

Hypersensitivities

As with all drugs, hypersensitive/allergic reactions and anaphylaxis may occur.

Reproductive

Menstrual irregularities, oligospermia, embryotoxicity, fetal deaths, abortion, and defective spermatogenesis.

Secondary Neoplasias

No controlled human data exists regarding the risk of neoplasia.

Miscellaneous

Back pain, chills, fever, and osteoporosis.

WARNINGS/PRECAUTIONS

- Deaths have been reported with the use of methotrexate in the treatment of cancer, psoriasis, and rheumatoid arthritis.
- Methotrexate has been reported to cause fetal harm, death, and congenital abnormalities. Males should avoid getting their partners pregnant during and for a minimum of 3 months after therapy and women for at least one ovulatory cycle. Pregnancy category D. It is not known whether the drug is excreted in human milk.

- Contraindicated in patients with known hypersensitivity to the drug, myelosuppression, severe renal and/or hepatic dysfunction.

SPECIAL CONSIDERATIONS

- Avoid aspirin, chloramphenicol, sulfonamides, tetracycline, phenytoin, and drugs, which bind to protein while on therapy.
- Refrain from folic acid and its derivatives during therapy.

Selected Readings

Bender JF, Grove WR, Fortner CL. High-dose methotrexate with folinic acid rescue. *Am J Hosp Pharm.* 1977;**34**:961-965.

Fisher RI, DeVita VT, Hubbard SM, et al. Diffuse aggressive lymphomas: Increased survival after alternating flexible sequences of ProMACE and MOPP chemotherapy. *Ann Intern Med.* 1983;**98**:304-309.

McRae MP, King JC. Compatibility of antineoplastic, antibiotic and corticosteroid drugs in intravenous admixtures. *Am J Hosp Pharm.* 1976;**33**:1010-1013.

Von Hoff DD, Penta JS, Hellman LJ, et al. The incidence of drug related deaths secondary to high dose methotrexate and citrovorum factor rescue. *Cancer Treat Rep.* 1977;**61**:745-748.

Von Hoff DD, Alberts DS, Mattx De, et al. Combination chemotherapy with cisplatin, bleomycin, and methotrexate in patients with advanced head and neck cancer. *Cancer Clin Trials.* 1981;**4**:215-218.

Mitomycin-C

MUTAMYCIN®, MITOMYCIN

MECHANISM OF ACTION

An antitumor antibiotic, mitomycin-C inhibits DNA synthesis, and at high concentrations inhibition of RNA synthesis may occur.

METABOLISM/EXCRETION

Clearance is affected by metabolism in the liver. Approximately 10% of the drug is excreted unchanged in the urine.

INDICATIONS

1. Adenocarcinoma of the stomach*, pancreas*, and colon
2. Advanced breast cancer

3. Non-small cell lung cancer
4. Ovarian carcinoma
5. Uterine cervix cancer
6. Cervical squamous cell carcinoma
7. Head and neck cancer

DOSAGE AND SCHEDULE

Adult

After full hematologic recovery (see manufacturer's guidelines to dosage adjustment) from any previous chemotherapy, the following dosage schedule may be used at 6-8 week intervals: 20 mg/m^2 IV as a single dose via a functioning IV. Because of the cumulative myelosuppression, patients should be fully reevaluated after each course of MUTAMYCIN, and the dose reduced if the patient has experienced any toxicities. Doses greater than 20 mg/m^2 have not been shown to be more effective and are more toxic than lower doses. See manufacturer guidelines for dosage adjustment based on nadir leukocyte and platelet counts.

No repeat dosage should be given until the leukocyte count has returned to 4000/mm^3 and a platelet count to 100,000/mm^3. When MUTAMYCIN is used in combination with other myelosuppressive agents, the dosage should be adjusted accordingly. If the disease continues to progress after 2 courses of MUTAMYCIN, the drug should be stopped since the chances of response are minimal.

Pediatric

Safety and effectiveness in children have not been well established.

ADMINISTRATION

Intravenous: Infuse slowly into the tubing of a freely running intravenous infusion of normal saline or D$_5$W. *Vesicant properties.*

STABILITY

Available in the lyophilized form in vials containing MUTAMYCIN 5, 20, 40 mg with mannitol 10, 40, 80 mg, respectively. Reconstituted mitomycin is stable for 14 days refrigerated or 7 days at room temperature. Mitomycin-C is purple in color.

DRUG INTERACTIONS
- Additive toxicity occurs in combination therapy with other myelosuppressive agents.

SIDE EFFECTS/TOXICITIES

Hematologic
Myelosuppression is delayed (4-8 weeks) and cumulative; recovery is usually within 10 days; septicemia and death can occur with severe leukopenia.

Gastrointestinal
Mild nausea and vomiting 1-2 hours and lasting up to 3 days; stomatitis is mild occuring within 5-7 days; anorexia, diarrhea, veno-occlusive disease (high doses).

Renal
Increases in serum BUN and creatinine; hemolytic uremic syndrome (HUS) (microangiopathic hemolytic anemia [MAHA], thrombocytopenia and progressive renal failure); this syndrome can include pulmonary edema, hypertension, and neurologic abnormalities; it can occur any time, have a delayed onset, and be dose-related.

Pulmonary
Dyspnea with a nonproductive cough, interstitial pneumonia. Chest x-ray may show infiltrates. Pulmonary toxicity occurs more frequently with cumulative doses ≥ 60 mg; acute shortness of breath and severe bronchospasm have occurred in patients who receive a vinca alkaloid and have received mitomycin-C in the past or are concurrently receiving mitomycin-C. FIO_2 concentrations greater than 50% perioperatively may induce adult respiratory distress syndrome in patients who received mitomycin with other chemotherapy combinations.

Cardiac
Congestive heart failure (rare).

Neurologic
Headache, blurring of vision, confusion, drowsiness, and syncope.

Dermatologic
Tissue necrosis and sloughing if the drug is extravasated; erythema and ulceration may be delayed

and occur at sites different from the injection site; increased sensitivity to sunlight; alopecia (mild), rashes, and purple-colored bands on nail beds.

Hypersensitivities

Acute shortness of breath syndrome; as with all drugs, hypersensitive/allergic reactions and anaphylaxis may occur.

Reproductive

Effect on the fetus and fertility is unknown.

Secondary Neoplasias

The drug may be carcinogenic.

Miscellaneous

Fever and fatigue.

WARNINGS/PRECAUTIONS

- Mitomycin-C is contraindicated in patients who had a hypersensitive or idiosyncratic reaction.
- Cumulative myelosuppression occurs with mitomycin-C. Manufacturer recommends dose reductions based on nadir counts. Withhold treatment with mitomycin-C until the WBC is $\geq$ 4,000/mm^3 and the platelet is $\geq$ 100,000/mm^3.
- Mitomycin-C is contraindicated in patients with hematologic disorders.
- Acute shortness of breath and severe bronchospasm have occurred in patients who receive a vinca alkaloid and have received mitomycin in the past or are concurrently receiving mitomycin-C. Onset within minutes to hours after the vinca alkaloid. Bronchodilators, steroids, and/or oxygen may be required to alleviate symptoms.
- FIO$_2$ concentrations greater than 50% perioperatively may induce adult respiratory distress syndrome in patients who received mitomycin with other chemotherapy combinations.
- Pregnancy category D. It is not known if the drug is excreted in human milk.

SPECIAL CONSIDERATIONS

- During administration of mitomycin patients should be asked to report any signs of pain, burning, or any other symptoms. Extravasation can occur in the presence of a good blood return and no complaints of pain or burning. Assessment of venous patency is required before, during, and after administration of mitomycin. In the event of extravasation, early intervention is required. The area should be examined frequently and a plastic surgeon consult should be considered.

- In patients receiving mitomycin-C with a vinca alkaloid, assess patients' tolerance to the last dose of treatment, any change may be an early indication of the acute shortness of breath and bronchospasm syndrome occurring.

Selected Readings

Chang AY-C, Kuebler JP, Pandya KJ, Israel RH, Marshall BC, Gormey DC. Pulmonary toxicity induced by mitomycin C is highly responsive to glucocorticoids. *Cancer.* 1986;**57:**2285-2290.

Crooke ST, Bradner WT. Mitomycin C: A review. *Cancer Treat Rev.* 1976;**3:**121-139.

Doll DC, Weiss RB, Issell BF. Mitomycin: Ten years after approval for marketing. *J Clin Oncol.* 1985:**3**(2):276-286.

Johnston-Early A, Cohen MH. Mitomycin C-induced skin ulceration remote from infusion site. *Cancer Treat Rep.* 1981;**65**(5/6):529.

Valavaara R, Nordman E. Renal complications of mitomycin C therapy with special reference to the total dose. *Cancer.* 1985;**55:**47-50.

Wood HA, Ellerhorst-Ryan JM. Delayed adverse skin reaction associated with mitomycin C administration. *Oncol Nurs Forum.* 1984;**11**(4):14-18.

Mitoxantrone HCl

NOVANTRONE®

MECHANISM OF ACTION

A synthetic anthracenedione (a new class of antineoplastic antibiotics), mitoxantrone HCl intercalates with DNA and inhibits topoisomerase II.

METABOLISM/EXCRETION

Mitoxantrone HCl is rapidly distributed to formed blood elements and tissues. High concentrations of the drug are found in the spleen, heart, and bone marrow. Excreted primarily through the hepatobiliary system and by a lesser extent the kidneys. Twenty-five percent of the drug is found in the feces and 6%-11%

is found in the urine after 5 days. Median half-life: 5.8 hours.

INDICATIONS

1. Acute non-lymphocytic leukemia (ANLL) including myelogenous, monocytic, promyelocytic, and erythroid acute leukemias (adults); used as remission induction therapy in combination with other agents*
2. Acute lymphoblastic leukemia
3. Chronic myelogenous leukemia
4. Advanced or recurrent breast cancer
5. Ovarian cancer

DOSAGE AND SCHEDULE

Adult

Combination initial therapy for ANLL: For induction, the recommended dosage is 12 mg/m^2 of Novantrone daily on days 1-3 given as an IV infusion, and 100 mg/m^2 of cytosine arabinoside for 7 days given as a continuous 24-hour infusion on days 1-7. Most complete remissions will occur following the initial course of induction therapy. In the event of an incomplete antileukemic response, a second induction course may be given. Novantrone should be given for 2 days and cytosine arabinoside for 5 days using the same daily dosage levels. If severe or life-threatening nonhematologic toxicity is observed during the first induction course, the second induction course should be withheld until toxicity clears.

Pediatric

Safety and effectiveness in children have not been established.

ADMINISTRATION

Intravenous: Usually given IV drip over approximately 15-20 minutes. Drug is diluted in 50 cc D$_5$W or normal saline and given with a free flowing IV infusion. The drug is not to infuse faster than 3 minutes.

STABILITY

Supplied as a sterile solution containing 2 mg/ml in multidose vials of 20 mg (10 ml), 25 mg (12.5 ml) and 30 mg (15 ml). Unused reconstituted solution should be discarded immediately, because it lacks a bacteriostatic additive.

DRUG INTERACTIONS
- Synergistic effects of cytarabine and mitoxantrone may exist.

SIDE EFFECTS AND TOXICITIES
Hematologic
Myelosuppression can be severe (dose limiting); leukocyte nadir in 10-14 days after treatment with recovery by day 21; anemia and thrombocytopenia.

Gastrointestinal
Nausea and vomiting (mild); mucositis 5-7 days after treatment (severity is dose dependent); diarrhea; elevation of liver enzymes.

Renal
Blue/green-colored urine may last 1-2 days; hyperuricemia.

Cardiac
Tachycardia, EKG changes (arrhythmias), chest pain, congestive heart failure, and a decrease in left ventricular ejection fraction (dose-limiting toxicity).

Neurologic
Seizures and/or headache.

Dermatologic
Increased sensitivity to sunlight, alopecia; a blue discoloration to the vein/skin may occur if extravasated; rare cases of tissue necrosis have occurred after extravasation.

Hypersensitivities
Allergic reactions: hypotension, urticaria, dyspnea, rash.

Reproductive
The drug has mutagenic and teratogenic properties.

Secondary Neoplasias
The drug may be carcinogenic.

Miscellaneous
Fever and blue discoloration of the sclera.

WARNINGS/PRECAUTIONS
- Cardiac toxicity may be more common in patients who have received prior anthracycline therapy, prior radiation therapy to the mediastinal area, and in patients with preexisting heart disease.
- Cumulative cardiac dose limit is 140 mg/m^2 in patients with no prior anthracycline therapy, no

cardiovascular disease, and no prior radiation therapy to the mediastinal area; 120 mg/m^2 in patients with prior anthracycline therapy.

- A decrease in the left ventricular ejection fraction (LVEF) by 25% is an indication to stop mitoxantrone HCl. Cardiac monitoring of EKGs and LVEF is recommended before treatment and at regular intervals.
- Patients with impaired hepatic functioning and/ or poor performance status may require a dose reduction. The safe use of mitoxantrone HCl in patients with hepatic insufficiency is unknown.
- Mitoxantrone HCl is contraindicated in patients with a prior hypersensitivity.
- Pregnancy category D. It is not known if the drug is excreted in human milk.

SPECIAL CONSIDERATIONS

- Treatment for tumor lysis syndrome should begin before treatment with mitoxantrone HCl with administration of allopurinol, alkalinization of the urine, and fluids.

Selected Readings

Arlin Z, Feldman E, Mittelman A, et al. High dose short course mitoxantrone (M) with high dose cytarabine (HIDAC) is safe effective therapy for acute lymphoblastic leukemia (ALL). *Proc Am Soc Clin Oncol.* 1991;**10**:223.

Crossley RJ. Clinical safety and tolerance of mitoxantrone. *Semin Oncol.* 1984;**11**(3, suppl 1):54-58.

Dorr RT. Antidotes to vesicant drug extravasations. *Blood Rev.* 1990;**4**(1):1-21.

Shenkenberg TD, Von Hoff DD. Mitoxantrone: A new anticancer drug with significant clinical activity. *Ann Intern Med.* 1986;**105**:67-81.

Weiss RB. Mitoxantrone: Its development and role in clinical practice. *Oncology.* 1989;**3**(6):135-141.

Paclitaxel

Taxol®

MECHANISM OF ACTION

A novel antimicrobial agent that promotes the assembly of microtubule formation and stabilizes them by preventing depolymerization. Paclitaxel is a dipertene plant product derived from the needles and bark of the western yew.

METABOLISM/EXCRETION

Majority of the drug is bound to plasma proteins (97.5%). Clearance of the drug is rapid. Hepatic and biliary excretion accounts for the majority of the clearance. Renal excretion is limited.

INDICATIONS

1. Metastatic ovarian carcinoma* (after failure of first line or subsequent chemotherapy)
2. Metastatic breast cancer
3. Non-small cell lung cancer
4. Metastatic melanoma
5. Gastric cancer
6. Acute leukemia

DOSAGE AND SCHEDULE

Adult

All patients should be premedicated before administration of Taxol to prevent severe hypersensitivity reactions. Such premedication may consist of dexamethasone 20 mg PO administered approximately 12 and 6 hours before Taxol, diphenhydramine (or its equivalent) 50 mg IV 30-60 minutes before Taxol, and cimetidine (300 mg) or ranitidine (50 mg) IV 30-60 minutes before Taxol.

Adequate trials of dose response have not been completed. Taxol at a dose of 135 mg/m^2 administered IV over 24 hours every 3 weeks has been shown to be effective in patients with metastatic carcinoma of the ovary after failure of first-line or subsequent chemotherapy. Larger doses, with or without G-CSF, have so far produced responses similar to 135 mg/m^2. Courses of Taxol should not be repeated until the neutrophil count is at least 1,500 cells/mm^3 and the platelet count is at least 100,000 cells/mm^3. Patients who experience severe neutropenia (neutrophil < 500 cells/mm^3 for a week or longer) or severe peripheral neuropathy during Taxol therapy should have the dosage reduced by 20% for subsequent courses. The incidence and severity of neurotoxicity and hematologic toxicity increase with dose, especially above 190 mg/m^2.

Pediatric

Safety and effectiveness in children have not been established.

ADMINISTRATION

Intravenous: Over 24 hours. Premedication required. Non-PVC administration sets should be used and an in-line filter with a microporous membrane not greater than 0.22 microns.

STABILITY

Solutions prepared as recommended by the manufacturer are stable at an ambient temperature (approximately 25°C) and lighting conditions for 27 hours. Prepared solutions may appear hazy.

DRUG INTERACTIONS

- Synergistic neurotoxicity may occur in patients receiving cisplatin and paclitaxel.
- Ketoconazole may inhibit the metabolism of paclitaxel.
- Increased myelosuppression may occur with the administration of paclitaxel after cisplatin.

SIDE EFFECTS AND TOXICITIES

Hematologic

Bone marrow suppression (dose limiting); severe neutropenia; median neutrophil nadir at day 11; thrombocytopenia (median platelet nadir day 8); anemia; fever associated with neutropenia.

Gastrointestinal

Mucositis (dose-related), diarrhea, mild nausea and vomiting; elevations in liver enzymes: bilirubin, alkaline phosphatase, and SGOT.

Pulmonary

Dyspnea.

Cardiac

Bradycardia (asymptomatic), hypotension, chest pain, arrhythmias, complete AV block, EKG changes (non-specific repolarization abnormalities, sinus tachycardia, premature beats).

Neurologic

Peripheral neuropathy (62% occurrence) is dose dependent; numbness, tingling and pain in the hands and feet; impairment of fine motor skills, difficulty walking, loss of deep tendon reflexes; arthralgia/myalgia manifested as pain in the large joints of the arms and legs is mild occurring in 2-3 days; grand mal seizures (rare).

Dermatologic

Alopecia; facial flushing during administration; paclitaxel is an irritant and may cause severe phlebitis if infiltrated into the subcutaneous tissue during administration.

Hypersensitivities

Hypersensitive reactions occur most frequently during the first 15-60 minutes of the infusion; reactions are not dose-related and can occur in patients without prior exposure to the drug. Reactions are thought to be histamine release-mediated and may be caused by the diluent Cremophor EL. Manifestations of severe hyper-sensitivity reactions include dyspnea with bronchospasm, hypotension requiring treatment, chest pain, angioedema (laryngeal stridor, epiglottic swelling, or periorbital edema), or generalized urticaria; death has occurred. Minor manifestations include dyspnea, flushing, rash, skin reactions, tachycardia, and hypotension.

Reproductive

The effect of paclitaxel on fertility has not been fully evaluated.

Secondary Neoplasias

The drug may be carcinogenic.

WARNINGS/PRECAUTIONS

- Premedication with corticosteroids, diphenhydramine, and H_2 antagonists is indicated before receiving paclitaxel to prevent severe hypersensitive reactions.
- For patients who experience severe hypersensitive reactions, discontinue the infusion and provide aggressive symptomatic treatment. Additionally, patients should not be retreated with paclitaxel. Minor hypersensitive reactions do not require discontinuing the drug.
- Contraindicated in patients with a history of hypersensitivity reactions to other drugs formulated with Cremophor EL.
- The development of significant conduction

abnormalities during paclitaxel administration may require treatment. Cardiac monitoring is required during subsequent cycles.

- Hematologic monitoring is required. Paclitaxel should not be initiated with a baseline neutrophil count of < 1,500 cells/mm³. Subsequent cycles should be held until the neutrophil count is > 1,500 cells/mm³ and platelet count is > 100,000 cells/mm³. A 20% dose reduction for subsequent courses is recommended for severe neutropenia (< 500 cells/mm³ for 7 days or more) during a course of Paclitaxel.
- Severe symptoms of peripheral neuropathy require a 20% dose reduction.
- Use cautiously in patients with hepatic impairment.
- Pregnancy category D. It is not known if paclitaxel is excreted in human milk.

SPECIAL CONSIDERATIONS

- Frequent vital sign monitoring is recommended during the first hour of the Paclitaxel infusion. Assess for anaphylaxis during infusion.
- The incidence of myalgias/arthralgias may be more frequent in patients receiving G-CSF after paclitaxel.

Selected Readings

Kris MG, O'Connell JP, Gralla RJ, et al. Phase I trial of Taxol given as a 3-hour infusion every 21 days. *Cancer Treat Rep.* 1986;**70**:605-607.

Rowinsky EK, Cazenave LA, Donehower RC. Taxol: A novel investigational antimicrotubule agent. *J Natl Cancer Inst.* 1990;**82**:1247-1259.

Rowinsky EK, McGuire WP, Guarneieri T, Fisherman JS, Christian MC, Donehauer RC. Cardiac disturbances during the administration of Taxol. *J Clin Oncol.* 1991b;**9**:1704-1712.

Sarosy G, Bicher A, Kohn E, et al. Patterns of G-CSF (G) usage in ovarian cancer patients receiving dose intense Taxol (T). *Proc Am Assoc Cancer Res.* 1992a;**33**:222.

Seidman A, Reichman B, Crown J, et al. Activity of taxol with recombinant granulocyte colony stimulating factor (GCSF) as first chemotherapy (C) of patients (PTS) with metastatic breast cancer (MBC). *Proc Am Soc Clin Oncol.* 1992;**11**:59.

Weiss RB, Donehower RC, Wiernik PH, et al. Hypersensitivity reactions from Taxol. *J Clin Oncol.* 1990;**8**(7):1263-1268.

Pentostatin

Nipent®, 2´-Deoxycoformycin, dCF, co-vidarabine

MECHANISM OF ACTION
Purine antagonist antimetabolite that interferes with
DNA replication and disrupts RNA processing. Cell
cycle nonspecific.

METABOLISM/EXCRETION
Ninety percent of the metabolites and unchanged drug
are excreted in the urine. Half-life: 5.7 hours.

INDICATIONS
1. Alpha-interferon-refractory hairy cell leukemia*
2. Chronic lymphoblastic leukemia
3. Mycosis fungoides
4. Acute lymphoblastic leukemia
5. Lymphoblastic lymphoma
6. Adult T-cell leukemia

DOSAGE AND SCHEDULE
Adult
Maximally active and tolerable dose is 4 mg/m^2/given
every other week after hydration with 500-1000 ml of
intravenous fluid, and followed by at least 500 ml.
Higher doses are not recommended.

Pediatric
Safety and effectiveness have not been established in
children or adolescents.

ADMINISTRATION
Administer *IV push* through the side port of a running
intravenous line. Verify venous patency before, during,
and after administration. Short (20-30 minute)
intravenous infusions (diluted in 25-50 ml of isotonic
solution) and *continuous infusion* therapy have been
utilized to administer pentostatin. Pentostatin is a severe
irritant.

STABILITY
Available in 10 mg vials. Reconstituted solution is
stable at room temperature for 72 hours. Dilution of the
10 mg vial with 500 ml of normal saline or lactated
Ringer's injection is stable for 48 hours at room
temperature.

DRUG INTERACTIONS

- The use of pentostatin concomitantly with fludarabine phosphate is not recommended because of the high number of severe and fatal pulmonary toxicities following this combination therapy.
- A hypersensitive vasculitis resulted in death in a patient receiving allopurinol and pentostatin; it is unclear if the death was a result of the combination.
- Combined use with vidarabine may potentiate the toxicity of each drug.

SIDE EFFECTS AND TOXICITIES

Hematologic
Severe leukopenia and thrombocytopenia; anemia is mild; ecchymosis and petechiae; granulocyte nadir 15 days; lymphocytopenia, both T and B lymphocytes are suppressed.

Gastrointestinal
Nausea and vomiting are mild to severe; anorexia; mucositis; rare hepatitis; mild elevation in SGOT.

Renal
Mild, reversible renal insufficiency (increased BUN and serum creatinine); hematuria and dysuria; hyperuricemia.

Pulmonary
Pulmonary infiltrates and nodules appear in patients with prior exposure to lung irradiation or bleomycin; cough, upper respiratory infection, bronchitis, dyspnea, epistaxis, rhinitis, sinusitis, pharyngitis, and pneumonia.

Cardiotoxic
Arrhythmia, chest pain, abnormal electrocardiogram, thrombophlebitis, and hemorrhage.

Neurologic
Lethargy, somnolence, seizures, mental confusion, headache, depression, nervousness, paresthesia, irritability; coma has occurred in 60% of patients.

Dermatologic
The drug is a potent irritant, avoid extravasation. Erythema, burning, tissue necrosis, and tissue sloughing; bacterial and viral skin infections; dry skin.

Hypersensitivities
Chills, pain, and fever; as with any drug severe allergic/hypersensitive reactions and anaphylaxis may occur.

Reproductive
The drug is teratogenic; adverse effects on human fertility have not been established; pentostatin can cause fetal harm.

Secondary Neoplasias
No carcinogenesis data are available.

Miscellaneous
Severe conjunctivitis (reversible with steroid eye drops).

WARNINGS/PRECAUTIONS
- Pregnancy category C. It is not known if pentostatin is excreted in human milk.

SPECIAL CONSIDERATIONS
- Hydration is necessary to ensure at least 2 l of urine output daily while on therapy.

Selected Readings

Foon KA, Nakano GM, Loller CA, et al. Response to 2´-deoxycoformycin after failure to interferon-alpha in non-splenectomized patients with hairy cell leukemia. *Blood.* 1986;**68:**297-300.

Grever MR, Leiby JM, Kraut EH, et al. Low-dose deoxycoformycin in lymphoid malignancy. *J Clin Oncol.* 1985;**3:**1196-1201.

Spiers AS, Moore D, Cassileth PA, et al. Remissions in hairy-cell leukemia with pentostatin (2'deoxycoformycin). *N Engl J Med.* 1987;**316:**825-830.

Procarbazine HCl

Matulane®, ibenzemethyzin

MECHANISM OF ACTION
Mechanism of action is unclear; it is thought to affect preformed DNA, RNA, and protein synthesis, cause chromosomal breakage, and inhibit methylation of transfer RNA. Cell cycle specific targeting S and G_2 phases.

METABOLISM/EXCRETION
Rapidly and completely absorbed from the GI tract.

Metabolized in the liver. Half-life: 1 hour. Seventy percent of the drug is excreted in the urine within 24 hours. Procarbazine crosses the blood brain barrier.

INDICATIONS

1. Hodgkin's disease* (MOPP regimen)
2. Malignant lymphomas, non-Hodgkin's lymphoma
3. Mycosis fungoides
4. Brain tumors
5. Small cell lung cancer
6. Multiple myeloma

DOSAGE AND SCHEDULE

The following doses are for administration of the drug as a single agent. When used in combination with other anticancer drugs, the Matulane dose should be appropriately reduced (e.g., in the MOPP regimen, the Matulane dose is 100 mg/m²/day PO for 14 days). All dosages are based on the patient's actual weight. However, the estimated lean body mass (dry weight) is used if the patient is obese or if there has been a spurious weight gain caused by edema, ascites, or other forms of abnormal fluid retention.

Adult

To minimize the nausea and vomiting experienced by a high percentage of patients beginning Matulane therapy, single or divided doses of 2-4 mg/kg/day for the first week are recommended. Daily dosage should then be maintained at 4-6 mg/kg/day until maximum response is obtained or until the WBC falls below 4,000/mm³ or the platelets fall below 100,000/mm³. When maximum response is obtained, the dose may be maintained at 1-2 mg/kg/day. Upon evidence of hematologic or other toxicity, the drug should be discontinued until there has been satisfactory recovery. After toxic side effects have subsided, therapy may be resumed at the discretion of the physician, based on clinical evaluation and appropriate laboratory studies, at a dosage of 1-2 mg/kg/day. Doses should be reduced in patients with compromised renal status and/or depressed hepatic function.

Pediatric

Use in children is not well documented and very close monitoring is mandatory. Undue toxicity, evidenced by tremors, coma, and convulsions, has occurred in a few cases. Dosage, therefore, should be individualized. The following dosage schedule is provided as a guideline only. Oral 50 mg/m²/day for the first week. Dosage should then be maintained at 100 mg/m²/day until maximum response is obtained or until leukopenia or thrombocytopenia occurs. When maximum response is attained, the dose may be maintained at 50 mg/m²/day. Upon evidence of hematologic or other toxicity, the drug should be discontinued until there has been satisfactory recovery, based on clinical evaluation and appropriate laboratory tests. After toxic side effects have subsided, therapy may be resumed.

ADMINISTRATION
Oral. Intravenous formulation is available for supervised investigational settings only.

STABILITY
Available in 50 mg capsules. Drug will decompose if exposed to moisture. Capsules are generally stable at room temperature for 2 years.

DRUG INTERACTIONS
- Drug interactions are well documented; we suggest a review of the literature for detailed descriptions of specific interactions.
- Contraindicated drugs include: ethanol, ephedrine, isoproterenol, epinephrine, tricylic antidepressants (imipramine and amitriptyline), paragylline, narcotic analgesics, antihistamines, phenothiazines, hypotensives, and barbiturates.
- Additionally, foods high in tyramine should be avoided (e.g., dark beer, wine, cheese, and bananas).

SIDE EFFECTS AND TOXICITIES
Hematologic
Myelosuppression, the most pronounced effect is thrombocytopenia with a nadir in 4 weeks, resolution in 4 to 6 weeks; leukopenia usually occurs after thrombocytopenia; patients with G6PD deficiency may develop hemolysis on oral procarbazine; increase in bleeding tendencies, purpura, petechia, and epistaxis.

Gastrointestinal
Nausea and vomiting occurs in the first few days of therapy, subsiding when tolerance develops; diarrhea

(protracted) or constipation, melena, abdominal pain, and anorexia may necessitate dose reduction; stomatitis, dry mouth, dysphagia; hepatic dysfunction, ascites, and jaundice.

Renal
Hematuria, urinary frequency, and nocturia.

Pulmonary
A rare, allergic-like pulmonary condition has been reported; pleural effusion, intercurrent infections (pneumonitis), and cough.

Cardiotoxic
Hypotension, tachycardia, and syncope.

Neurologic
Paresthesia, neuropathies, dizziness, ataxia, weakness, fatigue, lethargy, and headache, nightmares, depression, insomnia, nervousness, and hallucinations; tremors, convulsions, and coma less common.

Dermatologic
Alopecia, pruritus, dermatitis, urticaria, and allergic rash; rare hyperpigmentation, herpes, and flushing.

Hypersensitivities
Flu-like symptoms: fever, chills, sweating, myalgias, lethargy, and arthralgias most often occur with initial therapy; hypersensitive reaction defined as angioedema, urticaria, and a precipitous drop in serum complement.

Reproductive
Amenorrhea and azoospermia with high-dose procarbazine; gynecomastia and atrophy of the testes.

Secondary Neoplasias
Procarbazine is teratogenic, mutagenic, and carcinogenic.

Miscellaneous
Ophthalmic effects, nystagmus, diplopia, papilledema, photophobia, and retinal hemorrhages are rare; hearing loss, hoarseness, and slurred speech.

WARNINGS/PRECAUTIONS
- Contraindicated in patients with known hypersensitivity, thrombocytopenia, bone marrow depression, concomitant radiation.
- Caution should be observed in patients with renal and hepatic compromise.
- Patients should avoid alcohol while on therapy, for a

possible antabuse-like reaction.
- Patients should also avoid foods with known high tyramine content such as wine, yogurt, ripe cheese, or bananas.
- Pregnancy category D. It is not known if procarbazine is excreted in human milk.

SPECIAL CONSIDERATIONS
- Use nonphenothiazine antiemetics.

Selected Readings

Chabner BA, Sponzi R, Hubbard S, et al. High-dose intermittent intravenous infusion of procarbazine (NSC-77213). *Cancer Chemother Rep.* 1973;**57:**361-363.

Glovsky MM, Braunwald J, Opele G, Alenty A. Hypersensitivity to procarbazine associated with angioedema, urticaria, and low serum complement activity. *J Allergy Clin Immunol.* 1976;**57**(2):134-140.

Sponzo RW, Arseneau J, Canellos GP. Procarbazine-induced oxidative haemolysis: Relationship to in vivo red cell survival. *Br J Hematol.* 1974;**27:**587-595.

Streptozocin

Streptozotocin, Zanosar®

MECHANISM OF ACTION
An alkylating agent (nitrosourea), streptozocin inhibits DNA synthesis through intrastrand cross-linking of DNA. Cell cycle nonspecific.

METABOLISM/EXCRETION
Rapidly cleared from the plasma after administration (half-life 35 minutes). Drug metabolites cross into the cerebrospinal fluid. Drug concentrates in the liver and kidneys. Twenty percent of the drug is metabolized and/or excreted in the urine, and less than 1% in the feces.

INDICATIONS
1. Metastatic islet cell of the pancreas*
2. Carcinoid tumors
3. Non-small cell lung cancer
4. Squamous cell carcinoma of the oral cavity
5. Colon carcinoma
6. Hepatoma

DOSAGE AND SCHEDULE
Adult
Two different dosage schedules have been employed successfully with Zanosar.

Daily schedule:
The recommended dose for daily IV administration is 500 mg/m^2 for 5 consecutive days every 6 weeks until maximum benefit or until treatment-limiting toxicity is observed. Dose escalations on this schedule are not recommended.

Weekly schedule:
The recommended initial dose for weekly IV administration is 1,000 mg/m^2 at weekly intervals for the first two courses (weeks). In subsequent courses, drug doses may be escalated in patients who have not achieved a therapeutic response and who have not experienced significant toxicity with the previous course of treatment. However, **a single dose of 1,500 mg/m^2 should not be exceeded,** as a greater dose may cause azotemia. When administered on this schedule, the median time to onset of response is about 17 days and the median time to maximum response is about 35 days. The median **total** dose to onset of response is about 2,000 mg/m^2 and the median **total** dose to maximum response is about 4,000 mg/m^2.

The ideal duration of maintenance therapy with Zanosar has not yet been clearly established for either of the above schedules.

Pediatric
Safety and effectiveness in children have not been established.

ADMINISTRATION
Intravenous: Usually given IV drip over 15-20 minutes in D$_5$W or normal saline. Longer infusion times have been used. As a rapid bolus injection, intense pain and burning can result at the injection site.

STABILITY
Streptozocin in solution should be discarded after 12 hours because the product contains no preservatives.

DRUG INTERACTIONS
• Hyperglycemic drug interactions are possible.

- Use cautiously with steroids.

SIDE EFFECTS AND TOXICITIES

Hematologic

Myelosuppression is mild with a nadir in 1-2 weeks.

Gastrointestinal

Severe nausea and vomiting is more frequent with the daily dosage schedule; diarrhea; hepatic toxicity is manifested by an increase in SGOT, alkaline phosphatase, bilirubin, and hypoalbuminemia; jaundice.

Renal

Renal toxicity (severe and often fatal) is the dose-limiting toxicity; proteinuria (early sign), glycosuria, hypophosphatemia, azotemia, and renal tubular damage; nephrogenic diabetes insipidus.

Dermatologic

Pain and burning at the injection site during administration.

Hypersensitivities

As with all drugs, hypersensitive/allergic reactions and anaphylaxis may occur.

Reproductive

May adversely affect fertility.

Secondary Neoplasias

Secondary malignancies may occur after long-term therapy; acute leukemia has occurred. May be a carcinogen following topical exposure.

Miscellaneous

Altered glucose metabolism; fasting blood sugars may be elevated and a decrease in serum insulin levels have been seen; insulin shock and hypoglycemia.

WARNINGS/PRECAUTIONS

- Renal function must be monitored before, during, and after each course of streptozocin. Urinalysis should be done to detect early proteinuria.
- Blood urea nitrogen, serum creatinine, serum electrolytes, and creatinine clearance are recommended before, weekly, and at least 4 weeks after treatment.
- In patients with preexisting renal disease, the potential benefit of treatment to the risk of serious renal damage

must be taken into consideration.
- The use of other nephrotoxic drugs in combination with or concomitantly with streptozocin is not recommended.
- Patients should be monitored for hepatic or hematologic toxicity.
- Pregnancy category C. Nursing infants may experience serious adverse reactions from streptozocin.

SPECIAL CONSIDERATIONS
- Pain and/or burning during administration can be decreased or minimized by further diluting streptozocin, slowing the administration rate, and increasing the rate of the primary intravenous infusion.

Selected Readings

Gastrointestinal Tumor Study Group. Phase II studies of drug combinations in advanced pancreatic carcinoma: Fluorouracil plus doxorubicin plus mitomycin-C and two regimens of streptozotocin plus mitomycin-C plus fluorouracil. *J Clin Oncol.* 1986;**4**:1794-1798.

Kemeny N, Yagoda A, Braun D, et al. Therapy for metastatic colorectal carcinoma with a combination of methyl CCNU, 5-fluorouracil, vincristine and streptozotocin (MOF-Strep). *Cancer.* 1980;**45**:876-881.

Moertel CG, Douglas HO, Hanley J, et al. Treatment of advanced adenocarcinoma of the pancreas with combinations of streptozotocin plus 5-fluorouracil and streptozotocin plus cyclophosphamide. *Cancer.* 1977;**40**:605-608.

Moertel CG, Hanley JA, Johnson LA. Streptozocin alone compared with streptozocin plus fluorouracil in the treatment of advanced islet-cell carcinoma. *N Engl J Med.* 1980;**303**(21):1189-1194.

Weiss RB. Streptozocin: A review of its pharmacology, efficacy, and toxicity. *Cancer Treat Rep.* 1982;**66**(3):427-438.

Wiggans RG, Woolley PV, MacDonald JS, et al. Phase II trial of streptozotocin, mitomycin-C, and 5-fluorouracil (SMF) in the treatment of advanced pancreatic cancer. *Cancer.* 1978;**41**:387-391.

Thioguanine

6-Thioguanine, 6-TG, Tabloid® brand thioguanine

MECHANISM OF ACTION
Purine-based antimetabolite, inhibits de nova purine, DNA, and RNA synthesis. Cell cycle S specific.

METABOLISM/EXCRETION
Metabolized in the liver and excreted in the urine and feces. Oral absorption is incomplete and variable. Crosses placental barrier. Half-life: 11 hours.

INDICATIONS
1. Acute non-lymphocytic* and lymphocytic leukemias
2. Chronic myelogenous leukemia
3. Advanced colorectal cancer
4. Multiple myeloma

DOSAGE AND SCHEDULE
Adult and Pediatric
Tabloid brand thioguanine is administered orally. The dosage that will be tolerated and effective varies according to the stage and type of neoplastic process being treated.

On those occasions when single-agent chemotherapy with thioguanine may be appropriate, the usual initial dosage for adults and children is approximately 2 mg/kg/day. If, after 4 weeks on this dosage, there is no clinical improvement and no leukocyte or platelet depression, the dosage may be cautiously increased to 3 mg/kg/day. The total daily dose may be given at one time. The total daily dose is usually calculated to the nearest 20 mg.

Intravenous use is investigational; refer to primary literature sources for dosage information.

ADMINISTRATION
Oral: Total daily dose should be taken at once and between meals to facilitate complete absorption.
Intravenous: (Investigational) drip over 5-30 minutes in a minimum of 250 ml D_5W or normal saline.
Thioguanine is not a vesicant but care should be taken to assure venous patency to avoid extravasation. Large doses may be infused over 4 hours. *Continuous infusion* over 5 days is being evaluated.

STABILITY
Available 40 mg tablets. Store tablets at room temperature. Investigational in an injectable formulation, supplied as 75 mg in a 10 ml vial. Reconstituted solution is stable for 24 hours under refrigeration. Diluted

solution is stable for 24 hours under refrigeration or at room temperature.

DRUG INTERACTIONS

- Thioguanine increases the soft-tissue toxicity of busulfan.
- Cross-resistance exists with 6-mercaptopurine and Tabloid brand thioguanine.

SIDE EFFECTS AND TOXICITIES

Hematologic

Myelosuppression (dose-limiting), onset 1-4 weeks; with chronic therapy, myelosuppression may persist for several days after cessation of therapy; myelosuppression is $2^1/_2$ times greater with the intravenous formulation.

Gastrointestinal

Nausea and vomiting are dose-related and common in children only; anorexia and stomatitis (severe); diarrhea and severe stomatitis may warrant dose reduction; hepatotoxicity, with veno-occlusive disease (fatal in 2 cases), or jaundice (rare); esophageal varices in patients receiving thioguanine and busulfan.

Renal

Transient renal dysfunction, crystalluria, and elevations in serum creatinine and BUN; renal dysfunction can be serious and permanent; hyperuricemia.

Neurologic

Loss of vibratory sensation and unsteady gait.

Dermatologic

Pain and phlebitis if extravasated; rash, dermatitis, and dry skin.

Hypersensitivities

As with all drugs, hypersensitive/allergic reactions and anaphylaxis may occur.

Reproductive

May cause fetal harm and spontaneous abortions.

Secondary Neoplasias

The drug is mutagenic, teratogenic, and carcinogenic.

WARNINGS/PRECAUTIONS

- Contraindicated in patients with known hypersensitivity to thioguanine, prior drug resistance, liver disease, and myelosuppressed patients.

- Pregnancy category X. It is not known if thioguanine is excreted in human milk.

SPECIAL CONSIDERATIONS

- Doses may need to be reduced in patients with renal or liver impairment.
- Hyperuricemia can be minimized by increased urine alkalinization and the administration of allopurinol. Unlike mercaptopurine, thioguanine may be continued in the usual dosage when allopurinol is used conjointly to inhibit uric acid formation. The dose does **not** need to be reduced with allopurinol.
- Give oral doses on an empty stomach.
- Titrate dose if stomatitis develops.

Selected Readings

Griner PF, Elbadawi A, Packman CH. Veno-occlusive disease of the liver after chemotherapy of acute leukemia. *Ann Intern Med.* 1976;**85**:578-582.

Key NS, Kelly PMA, Emerson PM, et al. Oesophageal varices associated with busulphan-thioguanine combination therapy for chronic myeloid leukaemia. *Lancet.* 1987;**2**:1050-1052

Spiers AS, Kaur J, Galton DAG, Goldman JM. Thioguanine as primary treatment for chronic granulocytic leukemia. *Lancet.* 1975;**1**:829-833.

Thiotepa

Triethylenethiophosphoramide, Triethylene, TSPA, thio-TEPA, TESPA, Thio-Tepa

MECHANISM OF ACTION

Cell cycle nonspecific polyfunctioning alkylating agent. Chemically related to nitrogen mustard. Selectively reacts with DNA phosphate groups to produce chromosomal cross-linkage and blocking of nucleoprotein synthesis.

METABOLISM/EXCRETION

Rapidly cleared following IV administration; metabolized in the liver, with 60% excreted in the urine in 24-72 hours. Slow onset of action.

INDICATIONS

1. Adenocarcinoma of the breast*
2. Adenocarcinoma of the ovary*
3. Intracavity effusions secondary to diffuse or localized neoplastic diseases of various serosal cavities (pericardial, peritoneal, pleural)
4. Superficial papillary carcinoma of the urinary bladder*
5. Hodgkin's disease
6. Chronic granulocytic and lymphocytic leukemia
7. Bronchogenic carcinoma

DOSAGE AND SCHEDULE
Adult

Dosage must be carefully individualized. A slow response to thiotepa may be deceptive and may occasion unwarranted frequency of administration with subsequent signs of toxicity. After maximum benefit is obtained by initial therapy, it is necessary to continue the patient on maintenance therapy (1- to 4-week intervals). To continue optimal effect, maintenance doses should be no more frequent than weekly to preserve correlation between the dose and blood counts.

Initial and maintenance doses:

Initially the higher dose in the given range is commonly administered. The maintenance dose should be adjusted weekly on the basis of pretreatment blood counts and subsequent blood counts.

Intravenous administration:

Thiotepa may be given by rapid intravenous administration in doses of 0.3-0.4 mg/kg, given at 1- to 4-week intervals. For conversion of mg/kg of body weight to mg/m^2 of body surface or the reverse, a ratio of 1:30 is given as a guideline. The conversion factor varies between 1:20 and 1:40 depending on age and body build.

Intratumor:

Thiotepa in initial doses of 0.6-0.8 mg/kg may be injected directly into a tumor by means of a 22-gauge needle. A small amount of local anesthetic is injected first; then the syringe is removed and the thiotepa is injected through the same needle. The drug is diluted in sterile water for injection, 10 mg/ml. Maintenance doses at 1- to 4-week intervals range from 0.07-0.8 mg/kg depending on the condition of the patient.

Intracavitary:

The dosage recommended is 0.6-0.8 mg/kg. Administration is usually effected through the same tubing used to remove fluid from the cavity involved.

Intravesical:

Patients with papillary carcinoma of the bladder are dehydrated for 8-12 hours before treatment. The 60 mg of thiotepa in 30-60 ml of sterile water for injection is instilled into the bladder by catheter. For maximum effect, the solution should be retained for 2 hours. If the patient finds it impossible to retain 60 ml for 2 hours, the dose may be given in a volume of 30 ml. If desired, the patient may be positioned every 15 minutes for maximum area contact. The usual course of treatment is once a week for 4 weeks. The course may be repeated if necessary, but second and third courses must be given with caution since bone marrow depression may be increased. Deaths have occurred after intravesical administration, caused by bone marrow depression from systemically absorbed drug.

Pediatric

Safety and effectiveness in children have not been established.

ADMINISTRATION

Parenteral routes of administration are most reliable, since absorption of thiotepa from the GI tract is variable. Since thiotepa is a nonvesicant, intravenous doses may be given directly and rapidly without need for slow drip or large volumes of diluent. Some physicians prefer to give thiotepa directly into the tumor mass. This may be effected transrectally, transvaginally, or intracerebrally. For the control of malignant effusions, thiotepa is instilled directly into the cavity involved. *Intravenous push,* given as a rapid bolus injection via the side port of a running IV line. The drug is not a vesicant, but may act as an *irritant.* Pain and phlebitis should not occur at the injection site. *Intracavitary* administration is common; however, doses require further dilution to provide enough volume to be instilled. *Intramuscular, intravenous infusion,* and *subcutaneous* methods of administration may be used, but have no advantage over IV bolus. *Intratumor* (transrectally, transvaginally, intracerebrally) and *intraarterial* methods are also used.

STABILITY

Intravenous: 15 mg vials. Reconstituted vials are stable for 5 days. Thiotepa is compatible with D_5W, normal saline, dextrose/saline combinations, Ringer's injection, lactated Ringer's injection, procaine 2%, and epinephrine HCl 1:1000.

DRUG INTERACTIONS

- Increased apnea has been seen with concomitant use of succinylcholine.
- Myelosuppressive drugs potentiate hematopoietic toxicity.

SIDE EFFECTS AND TOXICITIES

Hematologic

Myelosuppression (dose-limiting); leukopenia nadir (7-10 days), fast recovery; platelets nadir in 3 weeks, can be delayed in onset and recovery.

Gastrointestinal

Nausea and vomiting are dose-dependent; onset in 6-12 hours after dosing; anorexia occasionally develops; stomatitis and ulceration of the intestinal mucosa.

Renal

Chemically-induced cystitis or hemorrhagic cystitis following intravesical administration is rare; it has not been reported following parenteral administration of thiotepa. A single case of renal failure has been reported. Hyperuricemia.

Pulmonary

Bronchoconstriction associated with an allergic reaction.

Neurologic

Dizziness and headache; parasthesias when administered intrathecally.

Dermatologic

Fever from a weeping subcutaneous lesion being treated; alopecia.

Hypersensitivities

Allergic reactions; hives, bronchospasm, and skin rash.

Reproductive

Amenorrhea (reversible in 6-8 months) and azoospermia; interference with spermatogenesis. Sterility may be reversible and incomplete.

Secondary Neoplasias

Thiotepa has mutagenic, teratogenic, and carcinogenic properties. Acute nonlymphocytic leukemia has been reported. A second breast cancer was seen in 36 of 633 women and solid tumors in 40 of 633. There have been a few reported cases on non-small cell lung cancer.

WARNINGS/PRECAUTIONS

- Contraindicated in patients with known hypersensitivity (allergy) to thiotepa, acute leukemias, existing hepatic and renal disease, severe bone marrow damage, concomitant radiation.
- Pregnancy category D. Thiotepa is excreted in human milk.
- Death and septicemia have occurred as a result of hematopoietic depression from thiotepa.
- Other drugs with known myelosuppressive properties should not be administered with thiotepa.

SPECIAL CONSIDERATIONS

- If WBC falls below 3,000/mm^3 and/or the platelet count falls below 150,000/mm^3, the dose should be discontinued.
- Administer allopurinol and sodium bicarbonate to maintain serum uric acid levels within normal range.

Selected Readings

Burnand KG, Boyd PJR, Mayo ME, et al. Single dose intravesical thio-TEPA as an adjuvant to cystodiathermy in the treatment of transitional cell bladder carcinoma. *Br J Urol.* 1976;**48**(1):55-59.

Pavone-Macaluso M. Permeability of the bladder mucosa to thio-TEPA, Adriamycin and daunomycin in men and rabbits. *Urol Res.* 1976;**4**(1):9-13.

Reimer RR, Hoover R, Fraumeni JF Jr, et al. Acute leukemia after alkylating-agent therapy of ovarian cancer. *N Engl J Med.* 1977;**297**:177-181.

Zarrabi MH, Rosner F, Grunwald HW, et al. Chronic lymphocytic leukemia terminating in acute leukemia. *NY State Med J.* 1991;**79**:1072-1075.

Vinblastine Sulfate

Velban®, VLB

MECHANISM OF ACTION

Vinblastine Sulfate is a vinca alkaloid derived from the periwinkle plant. It inhibits microtubule formation in the mitotic spindle, resulting in arrest of cell division at the metaphase stage. Cell cycle specific.

METABOLISM/EXCRETION

Rapid tissue binding to formed elements of the blood. Partially metabolized in the liver. Majority of the drug is excreted through the biliary system, 10% is found in the feces; 14% is found in the urine.

INDICATIONS

1. Hodgkin's disease* (Stages III and IV)
2. Lymphocytic lymphoma* (nodular and diffuse, poorly and well differentiated)
3. Histiocytic lymphoma*
4. Choriocarcinoma*
5. Mycosis fungoides* (advanced stages)
6. Advanced carcinoma of the testis*
7. Kaposi's sarcoma*
8. Letterer-Siwe disease* (histiocytosis X)
9. Breast cancer*
10. Bladder and renal cell carcinoma
11. Non-small cell lung cancer
12. Chronic myelocytic leukemia (blast crisis)
13. AIDS-related Kaposi's sarcoma

DOSAGE AND SCHEDULE

Adult and Pediatric

There are variations in the depth of the leukopenic response that follows therapy with Velban. For this reason, it is recommended that the drug be given no more frequently than *once every 7 days*. It is wise to initiate therapy for adults by administering a single IV dose of 3.7 mg/m^2; the initial dose for children should be 2.5 mg/m^2. Thereafter, WBC count should be made to determine the patient's sensitivity to Velban. A reduction of 50% in the dose of Velban is recommended for patients having a direct serum bilirubin value above 3 mg/100 ml. Since metabolism and excretion are primarily hepatic, no modification is recommended for patients with impaired renal function.

A simplified and conservative incremental approach to dosage *at weekly intervals* may be outlined as follows:

	ADULTS	CHILDREN
First dose	3.7 mg/m^2	2.5 mg/m^2
Second dose	5.5 mg/m^2	3.75 mg/m^2
Third dose	7.4 mg/m^2	5 mg/m^2
Fourth dose	9.25 mg/m^2	6.25 mg/m^2
Fifth dose	11.1.mg/m^2	7.5 mg/m^2

The above-mentioned increases may be used until a maximum dose (not exceeding 18.5 mg/m^2 for adults and 12.5 mg/m^2 for children) is reached. The dose should not be increased after the dose that reduces the WBC count to approximately 3,000 cells/mm^2. In some adults, 3.7 mg/m^2 may produce this leukopenia; other adults may require more than 11.1 mg/m^2, and very rarely, as much as 18.5 mg/m^2 may be necessary. For most adult patients, however, the weekly dosage will prove to be 5.5 to 7.4 mg/m^2.

When the dose of Velban that will produce the above degree of leukopenia has been established, a dose of *1 increment smaller* than this should be administered at weekly intervals for maintenance. Thus, the patient is receiving the maximum dose that does not cause leukopenia. *It should be emphasized that, even though 7 days have elapsed, the next dose of Velban should not be given until the WBC count has returned to at least 4,000/mm^3.* In some cases oncolytic activity may be encountered before leukopenic effect. When this occurs, there is no need to increase the size of subsequent doses.

The duration of maintenance therapy varies according to the disease being treated and the combination of antineoplastic agents being used.

ADMINISTRATION

Intravenously through the tubing or sidearm of a free-flowing intravenous infusion. Administer over approximately 1 minute. *Vesicant properties.*

STABILITY

Available in 10 mg vial. Solutions prepared with sodium

chloride injection (preserved with phenol or benzyl alcohol) may be stored in the refrigerator for 30 days. Protect from light. Preservative-free solutions used to prepare Velban must be discarded immediately.

DRUG INTERACTIONS

- Vinblastine in combination with other chemotherapy drugs may decrease the blood levels of phenytoin and increase seizure activity.
- Vinblastine may increase the cellular uptake of methotrexate by malignant cells.
- Vinblastine administered before bleomycin may enhance the effects of bleomycin.
- Raynaud's syndrome may occur with the combination of bleomycin and vinblastine.

SIDE EFFECTS AND TOXICITIES

Hematologic

Bone marrow suppression (dose-limiting); WBC nadir is in 5-10 days; recovery is within 7-14 days.
Thrombocytopenia is not as significant with recovery in a few days; anemia.

Gastrointestinal

Constipation, abdominal pain, paralytic ileus, anorexia, nausea and vomiting are mild; stomatitis, pharyngitis, hemorrhagic enterocolitis, diarrhea, and rectal bleeding.

Renal

Urinary retention (related to the neurotoxic effects); SIADH evidenced by a high urinary sodium excretion in the presence of hyponatremia.

Pulmonary

Acute shortness of breath and severe bronchospasm have occurred in patients receiving vinca alkaloids and more commonly in patients receiving vinca alkaloids in combination with mitomycin-C; onset may begin minutes to several hours after the vinca alkaloid; progressive dyspnea requiring chronic therapy may occur; vinblastine should not be readministered.

Cardiac

Hypertension, tachycardia, orthostatic hypotension; myocardial infarction and cerebrovascular accidents in patients receiving velban containing chemotherapy regimens (vinblastine, bleomycin, cisplatin) (rare).

Neurologic

Numbness of the hands and feet (parathesias), jaw pain, loss of deep tendon reflexes, peripheral neuritis, mental depression, headache, convulsions; cranial nerve paralysis.

Dermatologic

Alopecia, rash, photosensitivity, tissue sloughing if the drug is extravasated.

Hypersensitivities

As with all drugs, hypersensitive/allergic reactions and anaphylaxis may occur.

Reproductive

Amenorrhea and azoospermia.

Secondary Neoplasias

Patients treated with vinblastine in combination with other chemotherapy agents have developed leukemia (role of vinblastine is unknown).

Miscellaneous

Pain at the tumor site and muscle pain can occur after receiving vinblastine sulfate; the tumor pain can begin immediately and last a few hours; Raynaud's phenomena.

WARNINGS/PRECAUTIONS

- Intravenous use only. Intrathecal administration can result in death.
- An increase in the severity of side effects can occur in patients with impaired hepatic functioning or liver disease.
- The use of vinblastine is contraindicated in patients with bone marrow involvement who experienced a marked decline in the platelet and leukocyte count after a moderate dose of vinblastine.
- Contraindicated in patients who have significant granulocytopenia unless it is caused by the disease process.
- Vinblastine should not be used in the presence of bacterial infections unless the infection is under control before beginning therapy with vinblastine.
- Neurotoxicity may be more profound in patients with preexisting neurologic problems or in the weak and cachectic patient.
- The use of small amounts of vinblastine daily for long

periods is not advised.

- Pregnancy category D. It is not known if vinblastine is excreted in human milk.

SPECIAL CONSIDERATIONS

- Severe local tissue necrosis can occur if the drug is extravasated during administration. In the event of extravasation, stop administration of the drug immediately. Local injection of hyaluronidase and the application of warm compresses to the area will help disperse the drug and may minimize discomfort and the possibility of cellulitis.
- Prophylactic use of laxatives and stool softeners is recommended for all patients receiving vinblastine.
- Drugs known to cause urinary retention, particularly in the elderly, should be discontinued for the first few days after vinblastine.
- In patients receiving mitomycin-C with a vinca alkaloid, assess patient's tolerance to the last dose of treatment, any change may be an early indication of the acute shortness of breath and bronchospasm syndrome occurring.

Selected Readings

Bonadonna G, Zucali R, Monfardini S, DeLena M, Uslenghi C. Combination chemotherapy of Hodgkin's disease with Adriamycin, bleomycin, vinblastine and imidazole carboxamide versus MOPP. *Cancer.* 1975;**36**:252-259.

DiMaggio JJ, Kris MG, Gralla RJ, et al. Dose intensity versus toxicity trial in non-small cell lung cancer (NSCLC) with MVP [mitomycin + vinblastine (V)] + cisplatin (P) (meeting abstract). *Proc Ann Meet Assoc Cancer Res.* 1988:29.

Einhorn LH, Donohue J. cis-Diamminedichloroplatinum, vinblastine and bleomycin combination chemotherapy in disseminated testicular cancer. *Ann Intern Med.* 1977;**87**:293-298.

Ginsberg SJ, Comis RL, Fitzpatrick AV. Vinblastine and inappropriate ADH secretion (letter). *N Engl J Med.* 1977;**296**(16):941.

Kris MG, Gralla RJ, Kalman LA, et al. Randomized trial comparing vindesine plus cisplatin with vinblastine plus cisplatin in patients with non-small cell lung cancer with an analysis of methods of response assessment. *Cancer Treat Rep.* 1985;**69**:(4):387-395.

Vincristine Sulfate

Oncovin®, VCR

MECHANISM OF ACTION

A vinca alkaloid derived from the periwinkle plant.
Vincristine inhibits microtubule assembly causing an
arrest of cell division at the metaphase stage of mitosis.
Cell cycle phase specific at the M and S phase.

METABOLISM/EXCRETION

Excreted primarily by the liver with approximately 80%
of the drug found in feces, and approximately 10%-20%
found in the urine. Vincristine is distributed to body
tissues and bound to formed blood elements.

INDICATIONS

1. Acute leukemia* (acute lymphoblastic leukemia)
2. Hodgkin's disease*
3. Non-Hodgkin's lymphoma* (lymphocytic, mixed-
   cell, histiocytic, undifferentiated, nodular, and
   diffuse types)
4. Rhabdomyosarcoma*
5. Neuroblastoma*
6. Wilms' tumor*
7. Multiple myeloma
8. Breast carcinoma

DOSAGE AND SCHEDULE
Adult and Pediatric

Oncovin is administered IV at *weekly intervals.* The usual
dose of Oncovin for *children* is 2 mg/m^2. For children
weighing 10 kg or less the starting dose should be 0.05
mg/kg, administered once a week. The usual dose of
Oncovin for *adults* is 1.4 mg/m^2. A 50% reduction in the
dose of Oncovin is recommended for patients having a
direct serum bilirubin value above 3 mg/100 ml.

*Oncovin should not be given to patients while they
are receiving radiation therapy through ports that
include the liver.*

ADMINISTRATION

Intravenous: Infuse slowly (over approximately 1
minute) into the tubing or sidearm of a free flowing
intravenous solution. *Vesicant properties.*

STABILITY

Vincristine is light-sensitive; protect from light. Drug
must be refrigerated.

DRUG INTERACTIONS

- When used in combination with L-asparaginase (L-ASP), vincristine should be administered at least 12-24 hours before the enzyme. L-ASP administered before vincristine may decrease the vincristine clearance.
- Vincristine in combination with other chemotherapy drugs may decrease the blood levels of phenytoin and increase seizure activity.
- Vincristine may increase the cellular uptake of methotrexate.

SIDE EFFECTS AND TOXICITIES

Hematologic

Anemia, leukopenia, and thrombocytopenia (mild) nadir
10-14 days.

Gastrointestinal

Constipation, paralytic ileus; intestinal necrosis and/or
perforation; mucositis, anorexia, weight loss, diarrhea;
nausea and vomiting is minimal.

Renal

Polyuria, dysuria, and urinary retention; hyponatremia,
related to the SIADH.

Pulmonary

Acute shortness of breath and severe bronchospasm
occur in patients receiving vinca alkaloids; are more
common in patients receiving vinca alkaloids in
combination with mitomycin-C. Onset may begin
minutes to several hours after the vinca alkaloid.
Progressive dyspnea requiring chronic therapy may
occur; vincristine should not be readministered.

Cardiac

Hypotension and hypertension; coronary artery disease
and myocardial infarction have occurred in patients
treated with a vincristine-containing drug regimen and
have previously received radiation therapy to the
mediastinal area.

Neurologic

Dose-limiting toxicity; sensory, motor, and cranial

nerve functioning; sensory impairment and parathesia occur first, neuritic pain, motor weakness, loss of deep tendon reflexes, foot drop, difficulty in walking, ataxia, and paralysis all occur with continued treatment; paresis and/or paralysis of muscles (extraocular and laryngeal muscles most common) controlled by cranial nerves resulting in jaw pain, pharyngeal pain, parotid gland pain, and/or facial palsies; transient cortical blindness and optic atrophy with blindness; bone pain, myalgias, back pain, limb pain; convulsions followed by coma have been reported in children.

Dermatologic

Alopecia, rash, tissue necrosis if extravasated.

Hypersensitivities

Allergic/anaphylactic (rare).

Reproductive

Azoospermia and amenorrhea can occur in postpubertal patients, may be permanent; in prepubertal patients, permanency is less likely.

Secondary Neoplasias:

Secondary malignancies have occurred in patients receiving vincristine-containing regimens.

Miscellaneous

Fevers, headache, and fatigue.

WARNINGS/PRECAUTIONS

- Intravenous use only. Intrathecal administration can result in death.
- An increase in the severity of side effects can occur in patients with impaired hepatic functioning or liver disease.
- Vincristine should not be given to patients receiving radiation to fields that include the liver.
- Neurotoxic effects may be potentiated in patients with preexisting neuromuscular disease and/or in patients receiving other neurotoxic drugs.
- Vincristine may be held for signs/symptoms of neurotoxicity. Sensorimotor dysfunction may become progressively more severe with repeated doses.
- Paralytic ileus (may mimic "surgical abdomen") may occur, particularly in young children. Vincristine should be discontinued and supportive measures instituted.

- Pregnancy category D. It is not known if vincristine is excreted in human milk.

SPECIAL CONSIDERATIONS

- Extravasation of the drug can cause local tissue necrosis and cellulitis. In the event of an extravasation, stop administration of the drug immediately. Local injection of hyaluronidase and the application of warm compresses to the area will help disperse the drug and may minimize discomfort and the possibility of cellulitis.
- Drugs known to cause urinary retention, particularly in the elderly, should be discontinued for the first few days after vincristine.
- Prophylactic use of laxatives and stool softeners is recommended for all patients receiving vincristine.
- Monitor serum uric acid levels during treatment. Measures to prevent uric acid nephropathy should be instituted.
- In patients receiving mitomycin-C with a vinca alkaloid, assess patient's tolerance to the last dose of treatment; any change may be an early indication of the acute shortness of breath and bronchospasm syndrome occurring.

Selected Readings

Bain PG, Lantos PL, Djurovic V, et al. Intrathecal vincristine: A fatal chemotherapeutic error with devastating central nervous system effects. *J Neurol.* 1991;**238**:230-234.

Barlogie B, Smith L, Alexanian R. Effective treatment of advanced multiple myeloma refractory to alkylating agents. *N Engl J Med.* 1984;**310**:1353-1356.

Desai ZR, Van den Berg HW, Bridges JM, et al. Can severe vincristine neurotoxicity be prevented? *Cancer Chemother Pharmacol.* 1982;**8**:211-214

Holland JF, Scharlau C, Gailani S, et al. Vincristine treatment of advanced cancer: A cooperative study of 393 cases. *Cancer Res.* 1973;**33**:1258-1264.

Mauer AM, Simone JV. The current status of the treatment of childhood acute lymphoblastic leukemia. *Cancer Treat Rev.* 1976;**3**:17-41.

Bibliography

Baird SB, McCorkle R, Grant M, eds. Cancer nursing: a comprehensive textbook. Philadelphia: W.B. Saunders; 1991.

DeVita VT, Hellman S, Rosenberg SA. *Cancer principles and practice of oncology.* 4th edition. Philadelphia: J.B. Lippincott Co.; 1993.

Dorr RT, Von Hoff DD, eds. Cancer chemotherapy handbook, 2nd edition. Norwalk, Conn: Appleton & Lange; 1994.

Skeel RT. *Handbook of cancer chemotherapy.* 3rd edition. Boston: Little, Brown & Co.; 1991.

Wilkes GM, Ingwersen K, Burke MB. *Oncology nursing drug reference.* Boston: Jones & Bartlett; 1994.

Wilson BA, Shannon MT, Stang CL. *Nurses drug guide 1994.* Norwalk, Conn: Appleton & Lange; 1994.

CHAPTER 3

Management of Chemotherapy-Induced Side Effects

Chemotherapeutic agents are potent and have the potential to present many adverse effects. Toxicities and side effects are often a result of damage to dividing cells. Cells that are the most vulnerable by virtue of their rapid cellular division rate are cells found in the bone marrow, hair follicles, and gastrointestinal tract. Adverse effects range from mild to life-threatening. It is therefore critical for physicians and nurses to be knowledgeable regarding the drugs' adverse effects and the expected time of their occurrence.

A thorough patient assessment should be performed before administering any chemotherapeutic agent. A patient's tolerance to the prior dose of a given drug should be evaluated before administering the next course. Dose reductions or discontinuation of a particular drug may be warranted.

Patients and their families need to be educated regarding the potential side effects and their management, since many will occur when the patient is at home. In managing side effects, assessment and early intervention play a pivotal role in a patient's outcome.

GASTROINTESTINAL ADVERSE EFFECTS
Nausea and Vomiting
Nausea is defined as an unpleasant feeling, a wave-like feeling of distress, in the epigastrium, back of the throat, or throughout the abdomen. Nausea often precedes vomiting or retching.

Vomiting is the forceful expulsion of stomach contents through the mouth. Vomiting is usually accompanied by the following physiologic manifestations: excessive salivation, tachycardia immediately before vomiting, bradycardia during the vomiting episode, and decrease in blood pressure, weakness, dizziness, pallor, and increased rate and depth of respirations.

Retching is defined as a strong involuntary effort to vomit; a spasmodic movement of the abdomen in which the individual attempts to vomit, but no stomach contents are expelled. Often referred to as "dry-heaves."

Despite major advances in emetic research in the past decade, the mechanism of chemotherapy-induced emesis is still not completely understood. The hypothesis exists that reflex-induced emesis is caused by a stimulation of various receptors in the central nervous system and gastrointestinal tract. Receptor areas responsible for the act of vomiting have been identified in the vomiting center found in the lateral reticular formation of the medulla. The chemoreceptor trigger zone (CTZ) also found in the area postrema of the medulla is sensitive to stimuli from both the blood and the cerebrospinal fluid. Chemotherapeutic agents and/or their metabolites may stimulate receptors in the CTZ such as dopamine and serotonin receptors. Neuroreceptors are also located on the vagal and splanchnic afferent nerve fibers found within the gastrointestinal tract. It is theorized that chemotherapy damages the small intestinal mucosal cells; serotonin is then released from the enterochromaffin cells, which activates the vagal and splanchnic nerve fibers, which in turn leads to the stimulation of the vomiting center and the CTZ. Antiemetic agents that block neuroreceptors may be the answer in the prevention and control of chemotherapy-induced nausea and vomiting. Among the best studied and most effective agents in the prevention of chemotherapy-induced nausea and vomiting are those agents that block dopamine and/or serotonin receptors.

Three distinct patterns/phases of emesis have been identified in patients receiving antineoplastic agents.

Acute emesis occurs in the first 24 hours following exposure to emetogenic chemotherapy. *Delayed emesis* begins or persists for more than 24 hours after chemotherapy, is most often associated with cisplatin, and may persist up to 5 days after therapy. Delayed emesis has also been shown to occur following combinations of cyclophosphamide and doxorubicin. The mechanisms underlying delayed emesis have not been defined and may be different from those of acute emesis. The combination regimens of oral dexamethasone (8 mg BID for 2 days, then 4 mg BID for 2 days) with oral metoclopramide (0.5 mg/kg QID for 4 days) and oral dexamethasone (8 mg BID for 2 days, then 4 mg BID for 2 days) with prochlorperazine spansules (15 mg TID for 4 days) are effective antiemetic regimens used to treat delayed emesis induced by high-dose cisplatin therapy. With either regimen, treatment should be started the morning after chemotherapy and continued for 4 days. *Anticipatory emesis* is a classic Pavlovian conditioned response that occurs in the patient who experienced poor control of nausea and vomiting with prior courses of chemotherapy. The best treatment for anticipatory emesis is prevention during a patient's first exposure to chemotherapy. Behavioral interventions such as relaxation, distraction, and guided imagery may be useful in the management of anticipatory emesis. Individuals with cancer may experience emesis for reasons other than chemotherapy, such as medications (especially narcotic analgesics), and tumor-related problems (intestinal obstruction and cerebral metastases). It is extremely important to assess possible causes of nausea and vomiting other than chemotherapy.

Certain chemotherapeutic agents and combination regimens are more likely to cause emesis than others. The emetogenic potential of chemotherapeutic agents ranges from mild to highly emetogenic. Table 3-1 lists several chemotherapeutic agents and their associated degree of emetogenic potential. It is important to consider that agents are rarely given alone and are most often given in combination. Dose, route, and schedule

Table 3-1 Emetogenic potential of chemotherapeutic agents[a]

HIGH	MODERATE	LOW
Cisplatin	Cyclophosphamide*	Methotrexate*
Dacarbazine	Cytosine arabinoside*	Mitomycin-C
Mechlorethamine	Anthracyclines*	Bleomycin
Dactinomycin	Carboplatin	Busulphan
	Nitrosoureas*	Chlorambucil
	Procarbazine	Melphalan
	Ifosfamide*	Hydroxyurea
		Etoposide*
		Fluorouracil
		Vinca alkaloids

[a]Based on empirical observations.
*Potential increases with higher doses.

Source: Tonato M, Roilla F, Del Favero A. Methodology of antiemetic trials: A review. *Annals of Oncology.* 1991 **2**(2):107-14. Reprinted with permission of Klower Academic Publishers.

of administration are critical components in considering the degree, intensity, onset, and duration of nausea and vomiting for each agent given alone or in combination.

Despite the fact that the mechanisms of chemotherapy-induced nausea and vomiting remain obscure, formal studies have identified several effective agents that prevent chemotherapy-induced nausea and vomiting. Several novel agents now under development have the potential to further lessen chemotherapy-induced vomiting with fewer side effects. Table 3-2 lists common antiemetic agents (generic and trade names), their routes of administration, effective dose ranges, and the side effects associated with the dosage and schedule used for antiemetic therapy.

Research in the prevention of chemotherapy-induced emesis in the last several years has led a move from traditional single agent antiemetic therapy to the use of combination therapy and a new class of agents—serotonin antagonists.

Table 3-2 Antiemetics commonly used for the control of chemotherapy-induced nausea and vomiting

SEROTONIN ANTAGONISTS

granisetron   Kytril™

IV 10 mcg/kg × 1

Adverse Events: Headache, asthenia, somnolence, diarrhea, constipation, fever

ondansetron   Zofran®

IV 0.15 mg/kg Q4H × 3, or 32 mg × 1; PO 8 mg TID × 3 days

Adverse Events: Headache, diarrhea, constipation, fever, transient increases in serum SGOT/SGPT

SUBSTITUTED BENZAMIDE

metoclopramide HCl   Reglan®

IV 2-4 mg/kg Q2H × 4 or PO 0.5-2 mg/kg Q3-4H

Adverse Events: Sedation, akathisia, acute dystonic reactions (increased incidence in patients < 30 years), diarrhea (high doses), dry mouth

PHENOTHIAZINES

prochlorperazine   Compazine®

IM 10 mg Q3-4H, IV 10-40 mg Q3-4H, PO 10 mg Q4-6H, Spansule 15-30 mg Q12H, PR 25 mg Q4-6H

Adverse Events: Sedation, akathisia, extrapyramidal reactions, dry mouth, orthostatic hypotension, blurred vision

chlorpromazine HCl   Thorazine®

IM, IV, or PR 12.5-50 mg Q4-6H

Adverse Events: Sedation, hypotension, dizziness, akathisia, extrapyramidal reactions, dry mouth

perphenazine   Trilafon®

PO 4 mg Q4-6H, IM or IV 5 mg Q4H, or 5 mg IVB followed by an infusion at 1 mg/hr for 10 hours; maximum dose 30 mg (inpatients) and 15 mg (outpatients) in 24 hours

Adverse Events: Sedation, constipation, extrapyramidal reactions, dry mouth, rash

thiethylperazine maleate   Torecan®   Norazine®

IM, PO, or PR 10 mg QD-TID

Adverse Events: Drowsiness, extrapyramidal side effects (dystonia, torticollis, akathisia, gait disturbances), hypotension

CORTICOSTEROIDS

dexamethasone   Decadron®   Hexadrol®

IV 4-20 mg (10-20 mg given × 1, otherwise Q4-6H),
PO 4-8 mg Q4H × 4 doses

Adverse Events: Dyspepsia, hiccoughs, increased appetite,
euphoria, insomnia, flushing, fluid retention,
hyperglycemia

BUTYROPHENONES

haloperidol   Haldol®

IM or PO 2-5 mg Q2H × 3-4 doses, IV 2 mg × 1

Adverse Events: Sedation, akathisia, extrapyramidal reactions,
orthostatic hypotension

droperidol   Inapsine®

IM or IV 2-5 mg Q4-6H or drip

Adverse Events: Sedation, akathisia, extrapyramidal reactions,
hypotension

CANNABINOID

dronabinol   Marinol®

PO 2.5-10 mg 1-3 hours prior to chemotherapy, then Q2H × 4-6
doses/day

Adverse Events: Sedation, dry mouth, euphoria or dyphoria,
dizziness, orthostatic hypotension

ANTICHOLINERGIC

scopolamine   Transderm Scop®

Patch 0.5 mg/24 hours (1.5 mg over 3 days)

Adverse Events: Dry mouth, sedation, blurred vision,
mydriasis, restlessness

DRUGS USED TO AUGMENT ANTIEMETICS

diphenhydramine   Benadryl®

PO or IV 25-50 mg Q4H PRN

Adverse Events: Sedation, dizziness, blurred vision/diplopia,
dry mouth

lorazepam   Ativan®

IV 1-2 mg/m^2 × 1, not exceeding 3 mg; PO or SL 0.5-2 mg

Adverse Events: Sedation, anterograde amnesia, dizziness,
weakness, unsteadiness, disorientation,
hypotension

The concepts involved in the rationale for combination therapy include a more effective blockade of receptor sites; blockage of multiple receptor sites, blockage of receptor sites in different anatomic sites; a lessening of the side effects of chemotherapy, antiemetics, and cancer; a less cumbersome delivery; suitability for outpatient use; and reduced cost. Corticosteroids are commonly added to other antiemetics in combination therapy.

The new class of antiemetics, serotonin antagonists, do not cause extrapyramidal reactions, which make them an excellent candidate for combination antiemetic therapy. The combination of a neurotransmitter receptor blocking drug and a corticosteroid is the current world standard for patients receiving emetogenic chemotherapy.

Antiemetics should be administered prophylactically to patients receiving chemotherapy with known potential for causing nausea and vomiting. It is extremely important to cover the onset, peak, and duration of activity of each chemotherapeutic agent given.

The following are a few nonpharmacologic measures that may be used to minimize the extent and severity of chemotherapy-induced nausea and vomiting.

The health care provider should instruct the patient to:
- Eat foods served cold or at room temperature
- Drink clear liquids in severe cases of nausea
- Sip liquids slowly
- Eat bland foods
- Avoid spicy hot foods
- Rinse mouth with lemon water
- Avoid sweet, fatty, highly salty foods
- Avoid foods with strong odors
- Avoid eating or drinking 1-2 hours before and after chemotherapy
- Eat light meals throughout the day
- Use distractions such as music, television, games, and reading whenever possible
- Listen to relaxation tapes before, during, and after receiving chemotherapy
- Employ visual imagery music therapy

- Sleep during intense periods of nausea
- Practice good oral hygiene

The health care provider should continually assess the patient's response to antiemetic therapy and adjust the regimen to obtain maximum effectiveness. Prevention of nausea and vomiting is a major goal in the management of patients receiving chemotherapy. Combinations of antiemetic drugs provide the best protection from both acute and delayed vomiting. The cost-effectiveness of antiemetic therapy justifies their use when compared with other therapeutic and supportive care drugs used in cancer patients. Antiemetic regimens are highly effective and safe.

Bibliography

Aapro MS. Corticosteroids as antiemetics. *Recent Results Cancer Res.* 1988;**108**:102-111.

Andrews PLR, Rapeport WG, Sanger GJ. Neuropharmacology of emesis induced by anti-cancer chemotherapy. *Trends Pharmacol Sci.* 1988;**9**:334-341.

Baltzer L, Pisters KMW, Tyson LB, Rigas JR, Potanovich LM, Kris MG. High dose ondansetron (OND) plus dexamethasone (DEX) for the prevention of vomiting in patients (PTS) receiving multiple day cisplatin (CDDP). *Proc Am Soc Clin Oncol.* 1992;**11**:400.

Carmichael J, Bessell E, Hutcheon A. IV granisetron vs. IV granisetron plus IV dexamethasone in the prophylaxis of emesis induced by cytotoxic chemotherapy. In *Antiemetic Control: Maximizing the Benefits.* Abstract Book European Conference Clinical Oncology. Jerusalem, Israel, November 1993:36.

Cassileth PA, Lusk EJ, Torri S, et al. Antiemetic efficacy of dexamethasone therapy in patients receiving cancer chemotherapy. *Arch Intern Med.* 1983;**143**:1347-1349.

Chin SBY, Kocuk O, Peterson R, et al. Variables contributing to anticipatory nausea and vomiting in cancer chemotherapy. *Am J Clin Oncol.* 1992;**15**:262-267.

Clark R, Kris M, Tyson L, Gralla R, O'Hehir M. Antiemetic (AE) trials to control delayed vomiting (V) following high dose cisplatin (DDP). *Pro Am Soc Clin Oncol.* 1986;**5**:257.

Fozard JR. Neuronal 5-HT receptors in the periphery. *Neuropharmacol.* 1984;**23**:1473-1486.

Gralla RJ. Antiemetic drugs for chemotherapeutic support: Current treatment rationale for development of newer agents. *Cancer Supplement.* August 15, 1992;**70**(4):1003-1006.

Hesketh PJ, Murphy WK, Lester EP, Gandara DR, Khojasteh A, Tapazoglou E, et al. GR38032F (GR-C507/75): A novel compound effective in the prevention of acute cisplatin-induced emesis. *J Clin Oncol.* 1989;**7**:700-705.

Hockenberry-Eaton M, Benner A. Patterns of nausea and vomiting in children: Nursing assessment and intervention. *Oncol Nurs Forum.* 1990;**17**:575-584.

Kris MG, Gralla RJ, Clark RA, et al. Incidence, course, and severity of delayed nausea and vomiting following the administration of high-dose cisplatin. *J Clin Oncol.* 1985;**3**:1379-1384.

Kris MG, Gralla RJ, Tyson LB, et al. Controlling delayed vomiting: Double-blind, randomized trial comparing placebo, dexamethasone alone, and metoclopramide plus dexamethasone in patients receiving cisplatin. *J Clin Oncol.* 1989;**7**:108-114.

Kris MG, Baltzer L, Pisters KMW, Tyson LB. Enhancing the effectiveness of specific serotonin antagonists: Combination antiemetic therapy with dexamethasone. *Cancer Supplement.* December 15, 1993;**72**(11):3436-3442.

Morrow GR, Hickok JT. Behavioral treatment of chemotherapy-induced nausea and vomiting. *Oncology.* 1993;**7**(12):83-89.

Roilla F, Tonato M, et al. Prevention of cisplatin-induced emesis: a double-blind multicenter randomized crossover study comparing ondansetron and ondansetron plus dexamethasone. *J Clin Oncol* **9**(4):675-678.

Tonato M, Roilla F, Del Favero A. Methodology of antiemetic trials: A review. *Annals of Oncology.* 1991;**2**(2):107-14.

Constipation

Smooth muscles of the gastrointestinal tract can be affected by the neurotoxic effects of certain chemotherapeutic agents resulting in decreased peristalsis or paralytic ileus, a condition that causes constipation, the irregular or infrequent passage of hard feces.

Management

- Assess patient's normal bowel pattern.
- Assess the presence and character of bowel sounds.
- Explain to patient that the chemotherapeutic agents can cause constipation.
- Assess patient's dietary habits.
- Include high fiber foods and plenty of liquids in diet.
- Explain to patient the need for high fiber foods and to drink plenty of liquids.
- Explain need for prophylactic stool softeners.
- Place patient on prophylactic stool softeners.
- Avoid the use of enemas and suppositories in the presense of leukopenia and thrombocytopenia.
- Encourage patient to exercise, (e.g., walk).
- Assess for signs and symptoms of constipation.
- Instruct patient on the signs and symptoms of

constipation and to contact health care professionals if constipation occurs.
- Assess for signs and symptoms of impaction.
- Obtain x-ray of the abdomen.
- Hold chemotherapeutic agents causing the constipation until patient has a bowel movement; dose reductions may also be required.

Diarrhea

Epithelial cells of the gastrointestinal tract can be destroyed by certain chemotherapeutic agents causing an inadequate absorption and digestion of nutrients resulting in diarrhea. Diarrhea is the passage of frequent stools that are soft or liquid in consistency.

Management

- Assess patient's normal bowel pattern.
- Assess the presence and character of bowel sounds.
- Explain to patient that the chemotherapeutic agents can cause diarrhea.
- Assess for signs and symptoms of diarrhea.
- Instruct patient on the signs and symptoms of diarrhea and to contact health care professionals if diarrhea occurs.
- Assess patient's dietary habits.
- Include low fiber, high protein foods and plenty of liquids in diet.
- Explain to patient the need for low fiber, high protein foods and to drink plenty of liquids.
- Avoid foods that irritate the gastrointestinal tract.
- Explain need for antidiarrheal agents.
- Place patient on antidiarrheal medications.
- Encourage rest periods.
- Assess for signs and symptoms of impaction.
- Assess fluids and electrolytes; replace as necessary.
- Assess skin integrity, especially rectal area.
- Institute skin care regimen to prevent breakdown and promote comfort.
- Hold chemotherapeutic agents causing diarrhea until the diarrhea has resolved; dose reductions may be required.

Stomatitis

Chemotherapeutic agents can damage the rapidly

dividing cells of the oral mucosa resulting in inflammation of the oral and intraoral soft tissue, which can progress to painful ulceration and infection.

Management

- Assess oral cavity before each treatment.
- Assess patient's oral hygiene routine.
- Institute frequent oral hygiene.
- Explain to patient that the chemotherapeutic agents may cause mouth sores.
- Assess for signs and symptoms of stomatitis, bleeding, infections.
- Instruct patient on the signs and symptoms of stomatitis, bleeding, and infections and to contact health care professionals if these signs and symptoms occur.
- Avoid use of improperly fitting dentures.
- Keep lips well-lubricated.
- Avoid the use of commercial mouth washes containing alcohol.
- Avoid substances that are irritating to the oral mucosa such as tobacco.
- Maintain good nutritional intake and drink plenty of fluids.
- Avoid foods that are irritating to the oral mucosa.
- Consider use of topical antifungal or antiviral agents for infection.
- Assess the need for topical or systemic analgesics and topical protective agents for painful ulceration.
- Instruct patient on use of these medications.
- Hold chemotherapeutic agents causing stomatitis until it has resolved; dose reduction may be required.

Anorexia

A decrease or loss of appetite can be caused by chemotherapeutic agents. The effects of chemotherapy on other systems of the body (nausea/vomiting, stomatitis, diarrhea, constipation, taste alterations) can also lead to anorexia.

Management

- Obtain baseline height and weight.
- Assess for changes in weight before each treatment.
- Assess nutritional intake.

- Assess likes and dislikes regarding food and fluids.
- Encourage small frequent meals containing foods that are pleasurable to the patient.
- Provide an environment conducive to eating.
- Provide adequate antiemetic coverage to minimize nausea and vomiting.
- Avoid noxious smells when eating or cooking.
- Encourage nutritional supplements that are high in protein and calories.
- Consider supplemental enteral or parenteral nutritional support.
- Assess for contributing factors and intervene accordingly.
- Assess for electrolyte imbalance and replace accordingly.
- Assess plasma protein and serum albumin levels.

Doses of chemotherapeutic agents are based on a patient's weight. Accurate documentation of weight before each treatment is necessary so that doses may be calculated accurately. The doses of chemotherapeutic agents may be further reduced in the severely cachetic malnourished patient.

HEMATOLOGIC ADVERSE EFFECTS
Thrombocytopenia

A decrease in the platelet count can result in bleeding caused by the effect of chemotherapeutic agents on the bone marrow.

Management

- Monitor CBC, especially platelet count, before and after chemotherapy. Dose reductions may be required based on platelet nadir. Chemotherapy should be given only when the platelet count is within normal limits.
- Determine approximate nadir of platelets from chemotherapy.
- Assess for signs and symptoms of bleeding.
- Institute bleeding precautions.
- Avoid aspirin and aspirin-containing products.
- Instruct patient on signs and symptoms of bleeding and how to contact health care professionals.
- Instruct patient when brushing teeth to use a soft tooth

brush or toothette and avoid use of dental floss.
- Instruct patient to use electric razor.
- Avoid use of enemas, suppositories.
- Encourage use of stool softeners.
- Avoid valsalva maneuver.
- Avoid blowing nose forcefully.
- Avoid invasive procedures.
- Apply pressure to venipuncture sites for 3 to 5 minutes or longer if bleeding does not stop.
- For females during menstruation, monitor peri-pad count.
- Consider use of birth control pill or progestational agents to prevent menstruation.
- Maintain safe environment.
- Administer platelet transfusions as ordered.

Leukopenia/Neutropenia

A decrease in the white blood cell count and neutrophil count is caused by the effect of chemotherapeutic agents on the bone marrow.

Management

- Monitor WBC and neutrophil counts. Dose reductions may be required based on neutrophil and/or white blood cell nadir. Chemotherapy should be given only when the WBC/neutrophil count is within normal limits.
- Determine approximate nadir of WBC/neutrophil count from chemotherapy.
- Administer growth factors as ordered, e.g., G-CSF.
- Assess for signs and symptoms of infection.
- Instruct patient on signs and symptoms of infection and to contact health care professionals.
- Maintain strict handwashing and teach patient and family the same.
- Encourage good personal hygiene.
- Avoid exposure to potential sources of infection.
- Avoid invasive procedures.
- Maintain integrity of skin and mucous membranes.
- Administer antibiotics as ordered.

Anemia

A decrease in circulating red blood cells is caused by the effect of chemotherapeutic agents on the bone marrow.

Management
- Monitor CBC, especially hemoglobin and hematocrit before and after chemotherapy.
- Determine approximate nadir of hemoglobin and hematocrit from chemotherapy.
- Assess for signs and symptoms of bleeding.
- Instruct patient on signs and symptoms of anemia and to contact health care professionals.
- Monitor vital signs, administer oxygen if necessary.
- Institute bleeding precautions.
- Assess ability to perform activities of daily living, encouraging rest periods.
- Maintain safe environment, assist patient as necessary to prevent episodes of dizziness, syncope, and fatigue.
- Transfuse with blood products as ordered.

CUTANEOUS REACTIONS

Specific chemotherapeutic agents may produce alterations in the integumentary system that may be generalized or localized at the IV site or along the vein. These reactions include alopecia, flare reaction, erythema/urticaria, hyperpigmentation, radiation recall, and photosensitivity.

Alopecia

Temporary loss of hair is the effect of chemotherapy on the hair follicle. Hair loss may involve thinning, partial, or complete loss of scalp and body hair.

Management
- Prepare patient for hair loss, reinforcing that hair loss is temporary.
- Provide an environment that encourages expression of feelings.
- Assess impact of hair loss to patient and effect on lifestyle.
- Encourage patient to express feelings over hair loss.
- Encourage patient to purchase a wig, scarves, and hats before losing hair.
- Use scalp tourniquet or hypothermia to prevent or decrease hair loss if medically indicated; explain that these interventions are not always effective; explain risk of scalp micrometastasis.
- Instruct patient to avoid excessive shampooing and

hair combing.
- Instruct patient to use mild shampoo and hair conditioner.
- Avoid excessive blow-drying of hair.
- Avoid use of chemicals on hair (e.g., permanents, hair sprays, and dyes).
- Encourage support groups such as American Cancer Society's "Look Good Feel Better Program."
- Remind patient that hair loss is temporary and that hair will regrow when chemotherapy is complete.
- Explain to patient that hair may come back in a different texture, color, and thickness.

Flare Reaction

Most often associated with the anthracyclines, a flare reaction may be caused by a localized histamine release along the vein. Symptoms may include erythematous streaking, urticaria, and pruritus.

Management
- Assess skin integrity before starting IV for drug administration.
- Use a large vein for drug administration.
- Assess venous patency before, during and after drug administration.
- Administer drug with a free-flowing IV of normal saline.
- Assess for signs and symptoms of drug infiltration. If signs and symptoms of flare reaction occur, rule out drug infiltration, apply hydrocortisone cream topically, continue to administer normal saline intravenously; signs and symptoms will gradually disappear, usually lasting less than 1 hour.

Erythema/Urticaria

Erythema and/or urticaria may be a generalized or localized response to the chemotherapeutic agent.

Management
- Assess skin integrity before administering chemotherapeutic agents.
- Use a large vein for drug administration.
- Assess venous patency.
- Assess for onset, pattern, severity, and duration of reaction.

- Severe reactions may be indicative of hypersensitive reaction to the chemotherapeutic agent and may require discontinuing the drug.
- Administer antihistamine or corticosteroids as ordered.

Hyperpigmentation

A generalized or localized response to chemotherapeutic agents, hyperpigmentation may involve: nail beds, skin over joints and pressure points, interphalangeal and metacarpal joints, mucous membranes, and along veins used for chemotherapy administration.

Management

- Know which agents can cause hyperpigmentation.
- Assess skin integrity before starting treatment.
- Inform the patient that hyperpigmentation may occur and will gradually disappear when treatment is complete.
- Assess impact of hyperpigmentation on body image.
- Encourage patient to wear loose-fitting clothing.
- Recommend wearing long sleeves and using nail polish.

Radiation Recall

The recall reaction on skin areas previously irradiated is caused by certain chemotherapeutic agents that are administered at the same time or after radiation. The skin reaction can include erythema, dry desquamation, vesicle formation, and wet desquamation. Skin may be permanently hyperpigmented.

Management

- Assess skin integrity.
- Be familiar with agents that can cause radiation recall.
- Inform patient that radiation recall may occur.
- Maintain skin integrity.
- Assess skin daily for reaction and signs of infection.
- Follow skin care regimen recommended by the radiation oncologist or nurse if patient is currently receiving radiation therapy. Include gentle cleansing with mild soap, patting skin dry. Apply mild moisturizer to prevent dryness and cracking of skin (only when radiation treatments are complete).

- Avoid products that contain perfume, deodorants, or powders.
- Avoid use of tape or adhesive dressings on skin.
- Avoid extremes in temperature.
- Obtain dermatology consult.

Photosensitivity

An erythematous skin reaction caused by exposure to ultraviolet light after treatment with certain chemotherapeutic agents, photosensitivity can lead to severe tanning or sunburn.

Management

- Be familiar with agents that can cause photosensitivity.
- Assess skin.
- Assess onset, duration, and severity of reaction.
- Caution patient that exposure to sun (ultraviolet light) can cause a severe sunburn.
- Use a sunscreen with an SPF of 15 or greater.
- Avoid prolonged exposure to sunlight.
- Instruct patient to wear protective clothing, wide brimmed hat, long sleeves and pants.
- Employ above measures even when in the shade.

ACUTE SHORTNESS OF BREATH SYNDROME

This syndrome can occur in patients who have received or are presently receiving mitomycin-C and have received and continue to receive a vinca alkaloid. Onset can occur within a 2-hour range of receiving a vinca alkaloid with or without the administration of mitomycin-C, although it usually affects patients who have received 2 to 3 doses of mitomycin-C and 6 to 11 vinca alkaloid doses. Symptoms include severe tachypnea and dyspnea, and may also include wheezing, rales, and rhonchi. Chest x-rays may show bilateral infiltrates and pleural effusions.

Management

- Be familiar with this syndrome and its potential occurrence.
- Assess patient for tolerance from prior treatment, especially any change in breathing including mild dyspnea.
- Obtain a thorough and accurate medical history.
- Educate the patient and significant others that this

syndrome can occur within 2 hours of treatment and to report any changes in breathing to the health care team.
- If the syndrome occurs, immediately institute supportive measures: administer oxygen therapy, bronchodilators, and corticosteroids; obtain chest x-ray, blood gases, EKG.
- Provide psychological support.
- Do *not* administer further doses of a vinca alkaloid after this syndrome has occurred.

Bibliography

Baird SB, McCorkle R, Grant M, eds. *Cancer nursing: a comprehensive textbook.* Philadelphia: WB Saunders; 1991.

DeVita VT, Hellman S, Rosenberg SA. *Cancer principles and practice of oncology.* 4th edition. Philadelphia: J.B. Lippincott; 1993.

Dorr RT, Von Hoff DD, eds. *Cancer chemotherapy handbook.* 2nd edition. Norwalk, Conn: Appleton & Lange; 1994.

Groenwald SL, Frogge MF, Goodman M, Yarbro CH. *Cancer nursing principles in practice.* 3rd edition. Boston: Jones & Bartlett; 1993.

McNally JC, Stair JC, Sommerville ET. *Guidelines for cancer nursing practice.* Orlando: Grune & Stratton, Inc. 1985.

Oncology Nursing Society. *Cancer chemotherapy guidelines: module I-IV.* Pittsburgh: Oncology Nursing Society; 1988.

Otto SE. *Oncology nursing.* St. Louis: Mosby; 1991.

Potanovich LM, Gallina EJ, Pisters KMW. Acute shortness of breath syndrome following vinblastine (VLB) or vindesine (DVA) in patients receiving mitomycin (MITO): Nursing assessment and management. *Onc Nurs Forum.* 1991;**18**(2):355.

Wilkes GM, Ingwersen K, Burke MB. *Oncology nursing drug reference.* Boston: Jones & Bartlett; 1994.

Wilson BA, Shannon MT, Stang CL. *Nurses drug guide 1994.* Norwalk, Conn: Appleton & Lange; 1994.

Yasko JM. *Nursing management of symptoms associated with chemotherapy.* 3rd edition. Philadelphia: Meniscus Health Care Communications; 1993.

Key to FDA Use-In-Pregnancy Ratings

The Food and Drug Administration's Pregnancy Categories are based on the degree to which available information has ruled out risk to the fetus, balanced against the drug's potential benefits to the patient. Ratings range from "A," for drugs that have been tested for teratogenicity under controlled conditions without showing evidence of damage to the fetus, to "D" and "X" for drugs that are definitely teratogenic. The "D" rating is generally reserved for drugs with no safer alternative. The "X" rating means there is absolutely no reason to risk using the drug in pregnancy.

CATEGORY	INTERPRETATION
A	**Controlled studies show no risk.** Adequate, well-controlled studies in pregnant women have failed to demonstrate risk to the fetus.
B	**No evidence of risk in humans.** Either animal findings show risk, but human findings do not, or, if no adequate human studies have been done, animal findings are negative.
C	**Risk cannot be ruled out.** Human studies are lacking, and animal studies are either positive for fetal risk or lacking as well. However, potential benefits may justify the potential risk.
D	**Positive evidence of risk.** Investigational or post-marketing data show risk to the fetus. Nevertheless, potential benefits may outweigh the potential risk.
X	**Contraindicated in pregnancy.** Studies in animals or human or investigational or postmarketing reports have shown fetal risk, which clearly outweighs any possible benefit to the patient.

Index

A

Act-D; *see* Dactinomycin-D
Actinomycin-D; *see* Dactinomycin-D
Administration of drug, 7-8; *see also* specific agent
Adrenal steroids in management of anaphylaxis, 17
Adria; *see* Doxorubicin
Adriamycin; *see* Doxorubicin
Adrucil; *see* 5-Fluorouracil
Adult, nomogram for body surface from height and weight of, 4
Alkeran; *see* Melphalan
Alkylating agents, extravasation antidote for, 12-13
Alopecia as side effect, 164-165
amethopterin; *see* Methotrexate
aminophylline in management of anaphylaxis, 14, 17
amsacrine, extravasation antidote for, 12-13
Anaphylaxis, management of, 14-18
Anemia as side effect, 163-164
Anorexia as side effect, 161-162
Anthracyclines, emetogenic potential of, 154
Anticholinergics as antiemetics, 156
Antiemetics, 155-156
    augmentation of, 156
Antihistamines in management of anaphylaxis, 17
Ara-C; *see* Cytarabine
Asparaginase, 20-25
    with Daunorubicin, 63
    with Vincristine, 146
L-Asparaginase; *see* Asparaginase
Assessment guidelines, prechemotherapy, 1-2
Ativan; *see* lorazepam

B

BCNU; *see* Carmustine
Benadryl; *see* diphenhydramine
BiCNU; *see* Carmustine
Blenoxane; *see* Bleomycin
Bleo; *see* Bleomycin
Bleomycin, 25-28
    emetogenic potential of, 154
    as irritant agent, 10
    with Methotrexate, 108
Body surface, nomogram for, from height and weight
    adult, 4
    children, 5
BSF; *see* Busulfan

Notes

Notes